D1536637

Lyme Disease and Modern Chinese Medicine

An Alternative Treatment Strategy Developed by Zhang's Clinic

Dr. Qingcai Zhang and Yale Zhang

Sino-Med Research Institute
20 E. 46th Street, Suite 1402
New York, NY 10017, USA

Published by Sino-Med Research Institute
20 E. 46th Street, Suite 1402
New York, NY 10170, USA
Tel: 212 573-9584 Fax: 646-640-2713
Web site: http://www.zhangclinicnyc.com
           http://www.sinomedresearch.org

Products information: HepaPro Corp.
Web site: http://www.hepahealth.com
           http://www.hepapro.com

Call 1-888-788-4372 toll-free
First Printing: March 2006
Second Printing: May 2015
Third Printing: March 2019
Library of Congress Cataloging-in-Publication Data
ISBN 0-96772131-8

This book describes protocols and provides detailed herbal phytopharmacological data. Based on this data, practitioners can choose appropriate herbal supplements for their clients; however, this book is not intended as a substitute for medical diagnosis and medical treatment for patients with Lyme disease. If you think that you may have Lyme disease, consult your physician or healthcare practitioner.

Lyme Disease and Modern Chinese Medicine
Includes index:
1. Lyme disease. 2. Modern Chinese medicine
3. Case Studies.   4. Clinical data.

Table of Contents

Preface

This small book is long overdue. For more than three years now, our patients and many alternative and complementary medicine practitioners have asked us to present our clinical experiences and protocols on our modern Chinese medical approach to the treatment of Lyme disease. This book is the answer to their request.

Practitioners schooled exclusively in traditional Chinese medicine or conventional Western medicine may at first have some difficulty with our approach, which is a blending of the best of both TCM and conventional WM. We ask these practitioners to keep an open mind.

Most of the information in this book has been published on our web site www.sinomedresearch.org. Readers can visit the site to keep updated on new developments in treating LD with modern Chinese medicine.

Acknowledgements

Our Chinese herbal treatment system for Lyme disease was developed under the encouragement of Dr. Andrew Weil, a world leader in complementary and alternative medicine. His popular web site www.drweil.com has referred many LD patients to us for complementary and alternative medicine (CAM). Dr. Weil's strong support is the greatest endorsement of the work we are doing. His philosophy of integrative medicine and self-healing is the main principle used in our research and development. Without his continuing support, we would not be able to serve so many LD patients.

We would also like to thank our patients, who have encouraged us to write this book. Their feedback has helped us to continuously improve our protocols. Also, to the many medical doctors who referred patients to us, we express our heartfelt thanks—in particular, Lyme disease specialists Joseph Burrascano, Jr., M.D., Kenneth Liegner, M.D., Richard Horowitz, M.D., Virginia Sherr

M.D., and Steven Harris, M.D. We have also learned a great deal from their published articles and clinical findings. Thanks to Ms. Robynn Harris for putting us in her LD information e-mail list and for her daily e-mails that help keep us updated on new developments in this ever-progressing medical field.

HepaPro Corporation (1-888-788-4372) in California has helped us develop and produce the high-quality herbal remedies we use in our practice, in addition to providing excellent customer service to our patients. Please accept our thanks.

Miss May Tong, a premed student at the University of New York, read the manuscript and gave us very useful suggestions. Finally, we express our thanks to our editor Heidi Nye, who also served as editor of my previous three books on AIDS and on hepatitis C. Her exemplary English skills and attention to detail have brought clarity and smoothness to our writing.

Chapter I
Chinese Medicine

I-1: Introduction to Traditional and Modern Chinese Medicine

"...healing is the birthright of every human being. It does not have to be put into people or imposed on them from without but, rather, gently encouraged."

Andrew Weil, M.D.

Since the modernization movement of Traditional Chinese Medicine (TCM) in the late 1950s, three major systems of medicine are now practiced in China: Western medicine, TCM, and integrative Chinese and Western medicine. We refer to the latter as modern Chinese medicine (MCM).

Acupuncture was the first TCM modality introduced to the Western world; therefore, most Chinese medicine practitioners in the West are considered acupuncturists. The mainstay of Chinese medicine, however, has always been herbology, and most of TCM literature pertains to the study and application of herbs in treating diseases and maintaining health. Acupuncture is generally used as a supportive therapy, whereas herbs are used to treat difficult illnesses.

I-2: Traditional Chinese Medicine

At more than 5,000 years old, traditional Chinese medicine (TCM) is a well-documented health and healing system. It is one of the predominant forms of medicine in China and the second-largest medical system in the world, with more than 1 million practitioners and more than 25 percent of all the earth's inhabitants as its patients. TCM has documented more than 12,000 plant species as herbal remedies and treats almost every disease defined by Western medicine.

Based on a balance between yin and yang forces, TCM sees disease as a deviation from this balance, which TCM treatment seeks to restore. TCM's diagnosis entails inspection, auscultation and olfaction, inquiring, and palpation to collect symptoms, which are then summarized by eight principles (external or internal, hot or cold, excess or deficient, and yang or yin). Its major treatment methods are herbology, acupuncture, *tui-na* (a mix of chiropractic and massage techniques), and *qi gong* (a form of meditation and energy work).

I-3: Modern Chinese Medicine

Modern Chinese medicine (MCM) is the simultaneous study and practice of TCM and Western medicine (WM) in the same medical settings by the same doctors for the same patients. MCM adopts TCM principles and philosophy, while utilizing WM biomedical scientific data and diagnosis and treatment principles. New terminologies have been created for the blending of TCM concepts with modern pathophysiology and phytopharmacology. Furthermore, MCM has developed new concepts, new therapies, and new remedies to treat intractable and newly defined diseases, such as Lyme disease and hepatitis C.

To treat Lyme disease, MCM uses a TCM principle, known as *fu zheng qu xie*, which has been applied for centuries to treat infectious diseases. Literally translated as "support the righteous and dispel the evil," this principle advocates "regulating immunity and enhancing health to eliminate the infectious pathogen." Both homeopathic and allopathic, *fu zheng qu xie* is a constitutional approach that emphasizes the immune system in fighting disease. Herbs and acupuncture are used to enhance the body's defensive capabilities. In comparison, WM's treatment strategy for LD is using antibiotics to eradicate the pathogen (dispelling the evil) without regulating the immunity (supporting the righteous). An integrative TCM and WM approach combines these strategies to maximize treatment efficacy; this is the focus of our research and our practice.

I-4: Chinese Herbology

Herbology, the hallmark of the Chinese medicine, uses single herbal remedies, such as *qing hao* (*Herba Artemisiae annuae*)'s active ingredient artemisinin, as well as herbal formulas, which are a combination of herbs. Some 1,800 years ago, the Chinese medical sage Zhang Zhongjin established principles for the composition of herbal formulas. Typically, they consist of eight to 12 herbs. Each herb has a role—emperor, minister, assistant, or servant. The first two are the herbs that are responsible for the treatment of the disease. Assistants are used to mitigate the possible side effects of the main herbs, and servants enhance the effects of the main herbs, allowing them to target specific organs or organ systems. Chinese herbal formulas, when used properly, have little to no toxicity.

A common criticism of therapeutic herbs is the variability in the plant species, growing locales, seasonal factors, and processing procedures. In short, herbal products are not consistent in potency and quality. In addition, pesticides, chemical fertilizers, and heavy metals might contaminate raw herbs. Decoctions made from raw herbs usually exhibit strong unpleasant odors and tastes, making ingestion difficult. In order to overcome these obstacles, MCM developed herbal products using phytopharmacological principles to extract and purify the active ingredients of the herbs. Quality can be controlled, contaminations avoided, and, most importantly, therapeutic potency standardized. Extracted active compounds are then put into capsules and tablets, thereby making dosing and ingestion convenient and pleasant.

The following are our guidelines for the herbal products used in our clinic:

❖ The active ingredient is identifiable.

❖ The potency is measurable.

❖ The therapeutic action is predictable.

❖ The clinical outcome is repeatable.

According to TCM, herbs used for infectious diseases are *qing re jie du zao shi*—heat-clearing, toxin-resolving, and dampness-drying. The development of our formulas for treating Lyme disease is rooted in this category, and the pharmacological actions of the active herbal ingredients have been thoroughly tested in microbial cultures, animal models, and clinical applications. Of key importance is the fact that our herbal ingredients are more potent than raw herbs and less toxic than the pharmaceuticals used by WM to treat Lyme disease.

Chapter II

Lyme Disease

Lyme disease occurs worldwide, with most cases in temperate regions, and is the most common tick-borne disease in the United States. The 19th-century German doctor Alfred Buchwald first recorded a LD-similar condition in 1883. It is possible that LD may have existed for more than a hundred years prior to 1981, when Burgdorfer identified the *Borrelia* spirochete bacteria found in the stomach of ticks, named *Borrelia burgdorferi* (*Bb*). [1] The disease is now referred to as either Lyme disease or borreliosis.

In the United States, the major LD epidemical areas are the Northeast, Midwest, and Pacific Coast. Canada, Europe, and some Asian countries have also reported cases. It is possibly the fastest-growing infectious disease in the U.S. Nationally reported cases have more than doubled in a decade—23,963 in 2003 from fewer than 9,000 in 1993. In China, LD was first reported in 1985 and has now been identified in more than 19 provinces [2] .

Ticks not only carry *Bb*, but many other pathogens; consequently, Lyme disease actually involves multiple pathogenic co-infections. *Bb* has many genospecies, which may cause different disease courses, symptom patterns, and varying treatment responses.

Clinically, LD can be classified into three stages: localized acute infection, early disseminated disorders, and late chronic disseminated Lyme disease. In our practice, we mainly treat patients in the third stage, especially those who have not responded to antibiotics and have seen organ damage.

Chronic LD is an extremely complex and recurrent illness that is still poorly understood. Common symptoms are primarily neurological and muscular-skeletal fever, fatigue, mental fog, cognitive problems, arthritis, fibromyalgia, cardiovascular problems, and malaise.

Central nerve system (CNS) damage occurs in the majority of LD patients and is due to direct injury from the bacteria, autoimmune-triggered vasculitis, which reduces blood flow to the brain and certain neurotoxins. CNS damage includes cognitive problems, mental fog, memory loss, inability to concentrate, cranial nerve palsy, nerve root inflammation, and meningitis. The damage can occur in any of the 12 cranial nerves, as well as in the peripheral nerves, resulting in weakness, tremors, cramping, spasms, pain, numbness, tingling, loss of sensation or increased sensitivity, loss of coordination, and poor balance.

Muscular-skeletal system damage manifests as arthritis and muscle ache, which are often misdiagnosed as rheumatoid arthritis. Fibromyalgia is another common complaint that occurs due to inflammation in the muscle tissue. Patients with arthritis often show raised erythrocyte sedimentation rate (ESR) and anti-nuclear antibody (ANA), and test positive for rheumatoid arthritis (RA) factor.

Other less common organ damage includes heart muscle inflammation (carditis), hepatitis, gastrointestinal infection, and pneumonia. Because LD mimics so many diseases, it has often been misdiagnosed as multiple sclerosis (MS), rheumatoid arthritis, and amyotrophic lateral sclerosis (ALS), among others. It is not uncommon that a final LD diagnosis is established only after the patient has seen several doctors. Most patients in our practice have already been diagnosed and have exhausted conventional treatment options.

LD symptoms are due to multiple-pathogen infections, which can have a devastating impact on the patient's health. Why chronic LD is so difficult to treat is likely due to the reactivation of other latent infections, such as herpes, or the reactivation of a dormant *Bb* cyst.

Because diagnostic tests for LD are not conclusive, many patients miss the early treatment period. This usually leads to a chronic and persistent condition and is a major reason why so many people are suffering from chronic LD. In addition, conventional antibiotics do not often cover the whole spectrum of pathogens and pathogenesis that typify LD and so do not provide the necessary comprehensive therapeutic effect.

II-1: *Borrelia burgdorferi* Infection

Borrelia burgdorferi (the Lyme spirochete) infection is mainly transmitted through tick bites, though an infected pregnant woman can transmit it to her fetus, and breast-feeding is also a possible route of transmission. Transmission via sexual contact has not been confirmed. There is no evidence that casual everyday contact can transmit the disease. Contact with a Lyme disease-infected pet seems to be safe, although there is a chance of being bitten by Lyme disease-carrying ticks. Other rare possible routes of transmission are blood products and organ transplantation. Some blood-feeding insects might also transmit the Lyme spirochete, but this has not been well-studied or -documented.

After the initial infective tick bite, the earliest physical manifestation usually occurs as an *erythema migrans* (*EM*), which appears at the site of the bite. The rash is large in size (5cm or bigger) and lasts weeks and sometimes even months. Many patients, however, do not develop *EM*. Although the rash is considered an early local infection, dissemination can happen very fast, sometimes within a few days. Thus, early diagnosis is very important, as curative treatment is much easier to achieve during the acute stage.

Bb disseminates via both tissue and the bloodstream, making its way into the cardiovascular, muscular-skeletal, and central nervous systems. In disseminated LD, the patient will exhibit systemic symptoms and signs, the most common ones being fatigue, malaise, headaches, body aches, fever, chills, sweating, lymphadenopathy (lymph-node swelling), and stomach discomfort, as well as symptom patterns associated with particular organ systems, such as severe migraine-like headaches, arthritis, and arrhythmia. The complications of hematogenous-disseminated LD include secondary skin lesions, skeletal-muscular inflammation, mild hepatitis, cardiac disease, and neurological abnormalities. Like syphilis, Lyme disease is a great imitator, mimicking the symptoms, signs, and complications of diseases of almost every body system. Thus, the list of symptoms becomes very long.

There are some special features of Bb that make LD especially difficult to treat. Generally speaking, anti-bacterial agents can kill bacteria only during its division period. Most bacteria divide every 20 minutes and can be eradicated in a couple of weeks. However, the Bb spirochete divides more slowly, approximately every 12 to 24 hours. Therefore, a longer treatment course is usually required for eradication. In addition, studies have found three forms of *Bb*: bacterial (spirochete), spheroplast (lacking a cell wall and thereby named L-form), and cystic (dormant). Conventional WM treatments are only effective in combating the bacterial form.

Moreover, *Bb* can transform into a cyst and reactivate at a later time. The cyst form of *Bb* is the most difficult to eradicate as it is only susceptible to anti-bacterial agents when it reactivates. Studies have found that even after intensive antibiotic treatment, cysts persist in some 80% of patients. Re-infection by new tick bites can also occur, since patients do not acquire immunity from previous infection.

When *Bb* infects a patient, it invades fibroblasts and lymphocytes, binds with the host's proteins, and triggers the secretion of cytokines and antibodies, which in turn causes inflammation. If the infection is not effectively treated during the acute stage, the *Bb* will be widely disseminated and become much more difficult to eradicate. One particular feature of the Lyme spirochete is that it can also become an intracellular infection agent. Therefore, the anti-bacterial agents used to treat LD must be able to penetrate the cell membrane to kill the bacteria. Some antibiotics are only available in extra-cellular spaces and, therefore, are not able to totally eradicate the bacteria.

In chronic LD, symptoms usually worsen over a monthly cycle. This may be correlated to the Lyme spirochete's replication cycle. Effective treatment will reduce the severity of these flare-ups.

II-2: Co-infections of Lyme Disease

Factors that make LD even more complicated are co-infections. Nearly every Lyme patient receives co-infections from multiple tick-borne pathogens. The "Lyme" tick also transmits *Babesia, Ehrlichia, Bartonella, Mycoplasma,* and some other less-common pathogens, such as flavivirus, which causes Powassan encephalitis, and Q-fever bacteria, *Francisella tularensis,* which causes tularenmia. In the Northeast, about 2/3 of LD cases are co-infected with babesiosis, a malaria-like disease. *Bartonella,* human monocytic ehrlichiosis (HME), human granulocytic ehrlichiosis (HGE), Rocky Mountain fever, and *mycoplasma* are also common co-infections. These concurrent co-infections usually result in a wide range of symptoms and clinical presentations, rendering diagnostic tests unreliable and effective treatment more difficult. These co-infections contribute to the development of chronic and persistent forms of LD, and they must be considered in the overall treatment strategy for LD. [3]

One of the most serious LD co-infections is babesiosis, also known as piroplasmosis, which is a domestic- and wild-animal infection caused by the protozoa *Babesia microti, B. divergens,* and other strains. A 1996 study found that 50% of the *Bb*-carrying ticks in Connecticut were also infected with *Babesia*. Once *Babesia* enters the human body, it multiplies in red blood cells, resulting in febrile hemolytic anemia and hemoglobinuria, manifesting flu-like symptoms such as shaking, chills, night sweats, fever, and, in rare cases, even death. Babesiosis' pathology closely resembles malaria. Clinically, patients with chronic Babesiosis are characterized by the insidious onset of fever and chills, severe headaches, dyspnea, dry cough, dizziness, sweating, myalgia, encephalopathy, and mild to moderate hemolytic anemia. Diagnostic tests are not definitive, though the following can be used as references: Complete Blood Counting (CBC), *Babesia* smear, antibodies (IgG and IgM), and polymerase chain reaction (PCR) of blood. Especially for those patients who don't respond to prolonged antibiotics, the possibility of babesiosis co-infection should be considered and treated accordingly.

Another frequently encountered co-infecting microbial is *Ehrlichia*, which infects and destroys white blood cells. According to the various types of WBC it infects, *Ehrlichia* causes HME and HGE. Lyme ticks carry this parasite at a high rate in the Northeast. Symptoms are similar to other co-infection pathogens: fever, malaise, headache, sweating, muscle ache, and low WBC count. In conventional Western medicine, it is treated with antibiotics. Our anti-Lyme spirochete formulas also combat this pathogen.

II-3: Diagnosis of Lyme Disease

Lyme disease is difficult to diagnose with currently available tests, which cannot conclusively establish the presence of the causative pathogens. When conducting a clinical diagnosis, history of tick bites, existence of bull's eye rashes (*EM*), blood tests, symptom-patterns, and the occurrence of Herxheimer's reaction have to be considered.

The following table lists the most common Lyme disease symptoms. The number of organ systems affected and the degree to which they are affected depend on the duration of LD infection, the virulence of the spirochete, existence of co-infections, and constitution of the patient.

Common Symptoms List

System	Symptoms and Signs
General	Fever, sweats, chills or hot flushing, fatigue, weakness, poor stamina, weight loss or gain
Central Nervous System	Mental fog; confusion; difficulty in concentrating, reading, writing, speech, and thinking; headaches

	and lightheadedness; forgetfulness and short-term memory loss; disorientation; mood swings; irritability; depression; insomnia or excessive sleeping; paralysis, hypersensitivity, or loss of sensation
Peripheral Nervous System	Twisted muscles or tremors; tingling, numbness, burning, or stabbing sensations; shooting pain (peripheral neuropathy); facial paralysis (Bell's palsy)
Sensory	Double or blurry vision, floaters, hypersensitivity to light, tinnitus, ear pain, hypersensitivity to noise, motion sickness, vertigo, poor balance
Muscular-Skeletal System	Single or multiple joint pain, stiffness, or swelling; muscle pain, spasms, or cramps
Cardiovascular System	Heart palpitations, irregular pulse, heart murmurs or valve prolapse, vasculitis, Raynaud's syndrome

Respiratory System	Chest pain or rib soreness, shortness of breath, excessive coughing, sore throat
Digestive System	Upset stomach, constipation or diarrhea
Reproductive System	Low libido, testicular pain, pelvic pain, menstrual irregularity
Urinary System	Irritable bladder or bladder dysfunction
Other	Hair loss, swollen lymph glands

The majority of patients experience symptoms concentrated in the CNS and muscular-skeletal systems. For diagnostic and monitoring purposes, it is highly recommended that patients keep track of their symptoms and treatment responses in a journal.

The blood tests for diagnosing LD include those for antibodies and pathogens; however, the accuracy and clinical reliability of these tests have not been adequately established. Antibody-based tests, such as enzyme-linked immunosorbent assay (ELISA), indirect fluorescent antibody (IFA), and Western blot, can only tell if the person has ever contracted the infection. They cannot distinguish the difference between an active infection and a previous infection that has been cleared. During the acute infection period, it will take more than six weeks for antibodies to appear in blood. By then, the patient is already at a high risk for developing chronic LD, especially if arthritic and neurological symptoms are seen. A quicker and more reliable diagnostic method is needed to help prevent a large percentage of patients from developing chronic LD.

Even in the later stages of infection, the results of antibodies tests are not conclusive due to their low specificity and sensitivity. Sometimes the majority of antibodies have combined with antigens (the pathogens), forming immune complexes. This results in insufficient amounts of free antibodies in the bloodstream to be accurately tested. An infected patient might also have a compromised immune system that is not able to produce enough antibodies in order to test positive. In a trial of 10,000 patients with LD diagnosis by culture or DNA, 36% falsely tested negative on Western blot tests. Even with a positive antibody test, doctors often make different interpretations of the same results.

The recently developed PCR test is designed to detect pathogens and tell whether they are still present in the body. Ideally, the test should be able to determine if the disease manifestation is an ongoing infection. However, because of its low sensitivity and specificity, the Food and Drug Administration (FDA) and the Centers for Disease Control (CDC) have not acknowledged its value as a diagnostic tool.

Without a reliable diagnostic test, it is also difficult to monitor response to treatment and to establish a treatment endpoint. This has led to controversy over length of treatment, especially when health insurance companies are involved. In our practice, the treatment course is mainly based on clinical manifestations. Most of our patients have already been diagnosed by their conventional doctors and the duration of treatment largely depends on the individual's symptomatic improvement over time.

Diagnostic Treatment

For a patient has been tested inconclusively and is suspected to have Lyme disease, some times we can do a "diagnostic" treatment to see whether he/she is infected. In order for a treatment to be used for diagnostic purposes, it must be without harmful effects and able to trigger typical reactions. MCM treatment is safe and can trigger a typical Herxheimer's reaction, so it can be used as a "diagnostic" treatment. When a patient responds with initial Herxheimer's reaction and continues to see improvement with ongoing treatment, we can assume he/she may have LD and the treatment should be continued for the whole course. If the typical response is not shown, further diagnosis methods should be used to determine the cause of illness.

II-4: Conventional Treatments for Lyme Disease

Conventional Western medical treatments mainly use antibiotics to eradicate infectious pathogens. Antibiotics have bactericidal (bacteria-killing) and bacteriostatic (bacteria-suppressing) effects. Modern Chinese medicine examines the effectiveness of Western antibiotics in order to find TCM herbs that have similar pharmacological actions. We also examine why WM failed in order to avoid the shortcomings of antibiotic therapies.

Acute LD is mainly treated with the oral antibiotics, such as doxycycline, amoxicillin, and zithromax over a period of four to six weeks. Unfortunately, the time of treatment is usually not sufficient, partly due to the CDC's categorization of LD as a short-term disease. Treatment with antibiotics can suppress most patients' symptoms and eradicate the bacteria in some patients; however, in many cases in which early dissemination has already occurred, the spirochete remains and LD becomes chronic.

For chronic LD, conventional medicine uses long-term antibiotics. Typically, a patient will take many kinds of antibiotics, either orally or intravenously, in rotation. The length of treatment may be a year or even several years. Even such an intensive regimen is not a guaranteed cure. Rather, the success or failure of long-term treatment is dependent on many factors:

1. The sensitivity of the bacteria strain to certain antibiotics. Different strains of same bacteria can have quite different responses to the same antibiotics. Therefore, the same protocol might work for one patient but not for another. The reason for this is the bacterial resistance to treatment, which is covered in the next chapter. When we search for herbal remedies, microbial sensitivity is a main guideline. The anti-microbial spectrums of the herbal remedies discussed in this book have been compared to that of antibiotics.

2. The degree of dissemination of the LD when the antibiotics treatment is started. The later the treatment is started, the more difficult it is to eradicate the LD bacteria. Because of the difficulty of early diagnosis, many patients lose their chance for early treatment. The longer the disease course, the longer the treatment course. But a long course of antibiotics is not only hard for the patient to tolerate, it can also result in complications such as fungal infections, liver enzyme elevation, gall stones, and kidney damage—all of which make chronic LD even more difficult to manage with conventional medicine. As of this writing, once a patient has lost his/her tolerance for antibiotics, conventional medicine does not have anything else to offer.

3. The virulence of the bacteria strain, the amount of bacteria transmitted during the tick bite, and the location of the bite. The severity of the disease is, in part, directly related to the virulence of the *Bb* strain. Since the severity of the strains varies greatly, use of antibiotics alone may not be enough to deal with chronic LD.

4. The transformation of the LD bacteria into a cyst or spheroplast (without a cell wall, known as the L-form). In such cases, antibiotics are ineffective. Moreover, when treatment is stopped, the infection is reactivated. Neither WM nor MCM have an answer for such difficult cases. How to prevent these dormant forms from occurring and how to treat those that do occur are important research topics.

5. The presence of autoimmune complications. The pathogenesis of chronic LD includes direct cell and tissue damage, which may induce the production of cytotoxic and inflammatory factors and the crossing of reactive (autoimmune) antibodies that cause autoimmune complications. In order to properly treat chronic LD, the treatment protocol must address all aspects of the pathogenesis; however, conventional WM uses antibiotics as a stand-alone treatment. This is obviously not sufficient to deal with the overall problems of chronic LD.

6. The antibiotics used for clearing the bacterial pathogens, which is an etiological factor in the LD disease. In the later stage of LD, the pathogenetic factors have more profound affects on the disease prognosis than the etiological factor. Only using antibiotics to deal with etiology are obviously insufficient in the late stages of LD. From the holistic viewpoint of MCM if a treatment protocol does not cover the whole picture of the pathogenesis of a disease, it will not be very effective.

See Chapter III-2 for a more thorough discussion of the shortcomings of stand-alone antibiotics treatment.

In regards to *Babesia* co-infection, WM employs anti-malarial medications. Initially, clindamycin and quinine sulfate combinations were used, which were not only ineffective, but also caused severe side effects. Currently, high-dose azithromycin and mephron combinations are used, though they require a long treatment course (about four months), costs reach into thousands of dollars, and side effects include diarrhea, rash, and vertigo. Though MCM also uses anti-malarial remedies, its herbal formulas have a shorter treatment course and are much safer, more effective, and less costly than their WM counterparts.

II-5: Lyme Disease as a TCM Syndrome

TCM considers LD as *bi zheng* (numbness or stagnation syndrome) or toxic dampness-heat, which has a symptom-pattern similar to water retention, MS, rheumatoid arthritis, vasculitis, peripheral neuritis, and encephalitis. Its CNS and neurological symptoms are categorized as the TCM syndromes of *jian wang* (forgetfulness) and *shen bin* (mental fog). LD also resembles symptoms of syphilis and leptospirosis, which were common spirochete diseases in the old days in China.

The TCM principle for treating infectious disease is *fu zheng qu xie*, which literally means "supporting the right (immunity) and expelling the evil (pathogens)." The goal is to eradicate the pathogens by enhancing immunity. The main LD treatment principles are heat-clearing, dampness-drying, and toxin-resolving. The herbal formulas that we developed for LD are based on these principles. Phytopharmacological data has been used to confirm the formulas' actions: anti-pathogen, immune-regulating, anti-inflammatory, and tissue-regenerating.

Chapter III

Why Chinese Medicine?

III-1: Spirochete Diseases in China

TCM has a long history of treating spirochete diseases such as syphilis, yaws, rat-bite fever, relapsing fever, and leptospirosis. Indeed, TCM has proven particularly effective during the chronic stages of these spirochetal infections. The knowledge and clinical experience of TCM in treating these diseases can be applied to the treatment of LD, especially when conventional WM proves not so effective.

In our practice, we have seen LD patients with concurrent hepatitis C infection and other liver diseases. A long-term antibiotic regimen is usually not an option for such patients, due to the potential damage antibiotics can inflict on the liver. In contrast, MCM treatments are generally well-tolerated and do not harm liver functions.

III-2: Conventional Medicine's Problems in Treating Chronic LD

The major reason why LD patients turn to alternative medicine is WM's inability to effectively treat the disease in many cases. From our clinical experience, we have noted the following as problematic in stand-alone antibiotics treatment:

1. The extensive worldwide use and abuse of antibiotics have resulted in antibiotic-resistant bacteria and made antibiotics as a whole less effective. According to the Union of Concerned Scientists, Americans consume 3 million pounds of antibiotics per year and another 27 million pounds are used in farm animals. This has encouraged the mutation of virulent strains of antibiotic-resistant bacteria. Consequently, we have seen patients using 10 or more types of antibiotics in rotation without effect. Moreover, the treatment course for each antibiotic is usually not long enough to kill the bacteria, thus further encouraging resistance.

2. Antibiotics are generally designed for short-term use, usually for a period of a few weeks. Because *Bb* divides slowly and transforms into a dormant cyst, and because of the wide dissemination of the spirochete in the chronic form of the disease, the treatment time for LD must be sufficient to eradicate all bacteria. This usually requires at least six months, sometimes longer. Long-term use of antibiotics, however, damages the liver, gall bladder, bone marrow, auditory system, and kidneys.

3. Antibiotics are extracted from fungi and can suppress bacteria; however, long-term use can also

encourage fungi growth and infections, including urinary-tract and vaginal yeast infections, as well as flora imbalances.

4. Antibiotics are chemical compounds with high molecular weights, which make them more difficult to penetrate the blood-brain barrier, and antibiotics are less effective if they are unable to effectively penetrate the BBB. Moreover, the majority of chronic LD patients we've seen have exhibited CNS damage.

5. Antibiotics are only effective in suppressing bacteria, but most cases of LD are composed of multiple co-infections. Therefore, it is very difficult to deal with non-bacterial pathogens, such as *Babesia* and *Mycoplasma*. The anti-microbial spectrum of antibiotics is not wide enough to deal with these non-bacterial microbials.

6. Antibiotics can be very expensive—up to several thousand dollars per week—and difficult to administrate, especially in the case of intravenous drips, catheters, and long hours of daily administration.

7. In chronic LD, the patient 's inadequate immune response—autoimmunity and deposit of circulatory immune complex (CIC), which causes vasculitis and arthritis—further complicates the disease course. Since antibiotics have no immune-regulatory effects, using

antibiotics alone to treat chronic LD is not sufficient to cover all areas of LD pathology.

The conventional medical community is well aware of the problems inherent in stand-alone antibiotics usage in LD. The following is a quotation from an article written by eminent LD specialists:

"Relapses following use of potent antibiotics and detection of the Lyme organism or its DNA following treatment likewise demonstrate an inability to completely eradicate the pathogen and permanently halt the pathologic process with current methods of treatment in some patients. This is a problematic situation because intensive antibiotic treatment is costly, ... and carries associated risk for the patient. ... For some patients, however, this may be the only presently available alternative to progressive neurologic deterioration. In view of this dilemma, the international biomedical research community must give high priority to the development of improved and /or alternate methods of treatment that can definitively cure persisting Bb infections responsible for neurologic and other manifestations of chronic Lyme disease". [4]

Many Chinese medicinal herbal formulas are composed of active herbal ingredients that are similar in nature to antibiotics. For example, *Coptis chinensis* is an herb commonly found in formulas for diseases that are described in WM texts as bacterial infections that are treated with antibiotics. The strategic WM principle for infectious diseases is to identify and eradicate the pathogen with anti-microbial drugs; however, misuse of this strategy has resulted in a worldwide crisis, namely, over the past 60 years, we have inadvertently conducted a transcontinental breeding program of antibiotic-resistant strains of bacteria. In stark contrast, antibiotic ingredients in TCM formulas in continuous use for thousands of years have not caused resistant strains because these formulas are well-balanced with ingredients that support the anti-infection actions of the pathogen-suppressing herbs.

Chapter IV

Modern Chinese Medicine Approach to Lyme Disease

IV-1: MCM Understanding of LD

Western medicine considers external intervention the decisive factor in healing. As such it is less concerned about regulating immune response and promoting the repair of damaged tissue than it is with eradicating the infectious agent (external cause) by antibiotics (external intervention). Therapies based on this model are usually effective in acute critical diseases and traumas in which external factors are so overwhelming that internal factors need a great deal of assistance. For chronic infections and long-term illnesses, however, the side effects of extremely powerful treatment agents usually render disease management difficult for most patients.

In contrast, TCM maintains that the deciding factor in the occurrence of an infectious disease is the body's immune response. This theory is called *zheng xu xie shi*, which translates as "body's resistance weakened while the pathogenic factor prevails." During flu season, for example, most people are exposed to the flu virus, but only some of them develop the flu. Similarly, in an LD epidemic area, many people are exposed to tick bites, but not everyone develops LD. TCM holds that the body's internal factors decide whether the disease occurs or not, and if it does, how severe the disease course will be. Internal factors also play a major role in fighting the infection and restoring health.

TCM maintains that pharmaceutical drugs and herbs can only help the body heal; they cannot usurp its self-healing function. Eradication of the infectious agent is mainly conducted by the body's internal defenses; medical treatment only helps to strengthen and encourage these defense mechanisms. Although this strategy is not as effective as WM in dealing with critical diseases and traumas, it is a slower, but gentler process that is better suited for chronic and debilitating illnesses, like chronic LD.

IV-2: MCM Herbal Protocols for Chronic Lyme Disease

Modern Chinese medicine is the integration of TCM and WM strategies. MCM uses WM's pathophysiological and pharmacological knowledge to guide its research into TCM treatment methods. In MCM, TCM protocols are used as a "blueprint," while modern clinical and phytochemical research is used to isolate specific compounds found in raw herbs to deal with modern clinical diseases. In LD treatment, TCM's holistic treatment principles are applied to all aspects of disease management.

The fundamental requirement of an effective protocol is that it should match the pathogenesis of the disease. In LD, the *Bb* and co-infection agents can cause direct damage to the infected tissue cells. Anti-*Bb* and other anti-infection agents should be used to eliminate the infecting pathogens, but they are not the only treatments. The body's inadequate immune response to the infection must also be addressed.

Treatment must also administer to the body's inadequate reactions and peripheral damage, such as lymph-cell's production of cytotoxic and inflammatory mediators, which cause cell necrosis and inflammation. Prolonged over-active inflammation can cause severe damage to various organ systems. Arthritis, fibromyalgia, and Lyme-related encephalopathies revealed by SPECT (single photon emission computerized tomography) scans are examples of inflammatory damage. For these reasons, anti-inflammatory herbal remedies are included in MCM protocols for LD.

Another key aspect of LD pathophysiology is the process by which *Bb* and co-infection pathogens cause cross-reactive antibodies, thereby initiating self-perpetuating autoimmune responses that create antibody and antigen complexes. When these circulating immune complexes (CIC) deposit in blood vessels, vasculitis (inflammation of the vessels) occurs. This in turn leads to reduction of blood supply to the brain and causes symptoms in the central nervous system, such as brain fog, cognitive problems, and depression. Peripheral vasculitis also reduces blood supply to the peripheral nerves and can cause peripheral neuritis. In some cases, these neurological changes may assimilate to multiple sclerosis. CIC deposits in the muscle cause fibromyalgia and arthritis in the joints, Raynaud's syndrome, and Sjogren syndrome. Therefore, suppression of autoimmune antibody production, removal of CIC, and promotion of blood infusion to LD-affected tissue are very important parts of the MCM protocol.

We developed our LD protocol using the strategies outlined above. So far, we have seen no evidence of resistance by bacterial strains. Moreover, our herbal remedies have shown low toxicity suitable for long-term use, an ability to suppress fungi overgrowth, penetration of the BBB, and a wide anti-microbial spectrum. Our overall strategy is to use immune regulatory and supportive treatment to strengthen the anti-pathogen actions of the body, suppress autoimmune antibody production, control prolonged inflammation, remove CIC, increase blood infusion to LD-damaged tissue, and promote tissue healing.

IV-3: MCM Anti-*Bb* and Co-Infection Treatment

For acute *Borrelia burgdorferi* infection with early diagnosis by localized Lyme rashes, but without systemic symptoms, we use Allicin Capsule and HH Capsule for four to six weeks. This treatment usually eradicates the infection and prevents advancement to the chronic stage. The antibiotics employed by WM to treat *Bb* are also effective during the acute stage of the infection.

For chronic *Bb* infection and co-infections other than *Babesia* (anti-*babesia* treatment will be discussed in Chapter IV-4), we have developed four herbal remedies: Allicin Capsule, Coptis Capsule, HH Capsule, and R-5081 Capsule. Allicin and HH are used together as the first line of treatment. If a patient can't tolerate or does not respond to the first line, then Coptis Capsule and R-5081 Capsule are used together as the second line. Other combinations of these four herbal remedies have also been used as a second line of therapy.

The advantage of using Allicin Capsule is its active ingredient, 2-propene-1-sulfinothioic acid, S-2-propenyl ester (*allitridi*), [5-8] which has a very small molecular weight, (162.27) allowing it to easily penetrate the BBB and thereby making it suitable for CNS infections. It has a very wide spectrum of anti-microbial effects; it is effective against bacteria, mycobacteria, fungi, protozoa, and certain viruses. The safety of allicin is very high and its therapeutic index (Ld_{50}/ED_{50}) is as high as 134.9. [9-19]

Allicin is the odor-creating, chemically unstable ingredient of garlic. Therefore, we use its chemical precursor *allitridi*, which is chemically stable and turns into allicin once it is metabolized in the body. Garlic is a very popular supplement, and one can find shelves of garlic products in health food stores. Most of these products, however, are so-called "odorless garlic," which renders it useless as an anti-infection agent. For those patients who cannot tolerate the odor of garlic, taking chlorophyll along with allicin can make the odor less offensive.

The active ingredients of both coptis (umbellatine) and HH (dodecane carboaldehyde, 3-oxo) have small molecular weights (336.37and 198.30, respectively) and a wide spectrum of anti-microbial effects. They are the most frequently used anti-infection herbs in Chinese medicine. Allicin, Coptis, and HH Capsules exhibit virtually no toxicity and can be used safely for long-term treatments. They have been effectively used for treating leptospirosis in China. [20-23] Because Allicin, HH, and Coptis Capsules all have wide anti-microbial spectrums, when used for anti-spirochete treatment, they can suppress fungi growth. Their wide anti-microbial spectrum also makes them suitable for treating LD co-infections such as *Bartonella*, *Mycoplasma*, and

Ehrlichia. Clinically, we usually use two anti-microbial herbal formulas concurrently to maximize therapeutic efficacy and to prevent the development of possible resistance.

R-5081 Capsule is a TCM formula that has been used for treating syphilis for hundreds of years. Even for late-stage syphilis, it exhibits a cure rate over 50%. [24]

We have treated many children with chronic LD. Dosage is adjusted according to age and body weight. A common symptom in children is headache due to CNS infections, which we treat with Puerarin Capsule.

Response to treatment varies from person to person, depending on factors such as duration of infection, severity of symptoms, co-infections, strength of immune response, steroid use during infection, age, body weight, digestive functions, and compliance to treatment. The length of treatment is at least six months. Patients with a very long infection history may need to follow an open-ended treatment course to keep them well.

We ask our patients to keep daily treatment journals that track symptoms and response. This journal can help determine the length and the endpoint of treatment, as laboratory tests are still unreliable. With no standard laboratory marker, elimination of symptoms is the only way to judge whether an endpoint has been achieved.

To provide a clear understanding of herbal usage in chronic LD treatment, we designed a flowchart (see the end of this Chapter) that outlines how these herbal treatments are used.

IV-4: MCM Anti-Babesiosis Treatment

For babesiosis, MCM uses anti-malarial herbal compounds, mainly Artemisia Capsule. The main active ingredient, *qing hao su,* or artemisinin, was originally extracted from the herb *qing hao.* New derivatives of artemisinin have shown greater efficacy, reduced relapse rate, and diminished toxicity levels. Artemisinin is no longer used clinically, since more effective and safer derivatives, such as artesunate, have become the standard treatment remedies.

Artemisinin was tested to be lethal to Endoerythrocytic plasmodium. Symptomatic control and negative plasmodium examination were achieved more rapidly by using artemisinin compared with chloroquine. [25-29] Compared with conventional treatment, Artemisia Capsule has a shorter treatment course, is much less expensive, and causes almost no side effects. The treatment course is around two to three months and it should be extended in cases of chronic infection. If babesiosis is diagnosed with LD, the former should be treated first, so that subsequent therapy for LD and other co-infections, such as *Ehrlichia*, will be more effective. Moreover, babesiosis treatment is much shorter and simpler than that for LD.

Artemisia has been shown to regulate immune function and has been used in treating lupus erythematous discoides (LED) and rheumatoid arthritis. [29a] Therefore, it can also be used in the treatment of autoimmune symptoms such as fibromyalgia, arthritis, and vasculitis. Recently, artemisia has been found to have anti-cancer effects by promoting apoptosis and has the potential to become a non-toxic supplemental anti-cancer treatment, though further research is needed.

IV-5: MCM Constitutional Supportive Treatments

When an infectious disease becomes chronic and persists for many years, the pathogenetic factors play a much more profound role than the etiological factors in the prognosis of a disease. During the chronic stage, focusing only on eradicating the pathogen is not sufficient.

In chronic LD, the following constitutional damage is often seen: demyelination and axon loss, small blood vessel vasculitis, blood hypo-fusion, ischemia, memory loss, sleep disorders, verbal and cognitive difficulties, CIC deposit, arthralgia, fibromyalgia, and cardiovascular disorders. These constitutional signs form the main symptom-pattern of chronic LD, which can persist even after the infectious agent has been eliminated.

Therefore, the third segment of the LD treatment deals with constitutional and supportive treatment, which is not emphasized in conventional WM. The focus of MCM constitutional treatment is to promote recovery from the cumulative damage caused by chronic LD, utilizing anti-inflammatory, microcirculation-promoting, phagocytosis-promoting (removal of CIC), and immune-regulating components to normalize health status and overall life quality.

Another reason to introduce MCM for treating these constitutional manifestations is that conventional treatment for them often conflicts with the treatment of underlying LD. Conventional medicine often uses steroids such as prednisone to suppress autoimmunity and inflammation. But this approach can further disseminate the *Bb* infection, making its eradication more difficult. MCM treatments do not have this problem.

MCM constitutional treatments include the following:

A). For patients with joint pain, muscle ache, fibromyalgia, skin rashes, allergies, vasculitis, Raynaud's syndrome, Sjogren syndrome, and severe Herxheimer's reaction, AI #3 Capsule should be used. It is designed to suppress autoimmune antibody production and to control inflammation. If these symptoms are severe, the dosage is five capsules per day—two in the morning, one at noon, and two in the evening. We recommend taking the capsules with food. Once the symptoms begin to subside, the dose should be reduced to one capsule, three times a day. When symptoms are relieved, AI #3 Capsule should be discontinued. This herbal remedy is used for suppressing humeral immunity and autoimmune reactions, and reducing inflammation. In conventional medicine, these autoimmune complications are typically treated with steroids. We have seen patients misdiagnosed as MS or rheumatoid arthritis and treated with steroids, which caused their LD symptoms to dramatically worsen and caused permanent damage. This kind of treatment conflict is not seen with AI #3 Capsule.

For joint pain and arthritis symptoms, Arthral EZ Tablet can also be used, at a dose of one tablet three times a day.

B). Fatigue is one of the most common complaints of LD patients. Cordyceps Capsule can be used to improve energy level and enhance immunity, especially cellular immunity. It is an important herbal remedy used in TCM for convalescence purpose. [30-34]

C). CNS symptoms, such as difficulty in concentration, depression, cognitive problems, and memory loss are usually caused by vasculitis, which reduces blood supply to the brain. Another possible cause is that *Bb* may produce neurotoxins that hinder brain functions. In order to increase blood infusion to the brain and remove neurotoxins, the underlying vasculitis must be treated by suppressing autoimmune antibody production and removing the CIC, using AI #3 Capsule and Circulation P Capsule. In addition, we also use Puerarin Capsule, which increases blood infusion to the brain, enhances brain functions, and improves the vasomotor mechanisms that can help alleviate headaches and migraines. [35]

D). If the patient complains of insomnia or restless sleep, HerbSom Capsule can be used. It is a gentle, effective, and non-addictive sleep aid that mainly induces relaxation and improves the quality of sleep. It will not cause drowsiness in the morning.

E). Circulation P Capsule is a necessity for all patients, since it increases blood infusion to the tissues, restores inflammation-damaged tissues, and promotes the phagocytosis activity of macrophages for the removal of deposited circulatory immune complexes and neurotoxins in inflamed tissues. [36-39]

IV-6: Herxheimer's Reaction

Both anti-spirochete and anti-*Babesia* herbal treatment may induce Herxheimer's reaction during the first few weeks of treatment. A Herxheimer's reaction is part of the immune system's response to the death of the spirochete or *Babesia*. Typically, symptoms will worsen temporarily, which indicates that the patient is responding to the treatment. If the reaction becomes too difficult to tolerate, then dosage of herbs should be reduced to half or even less, and gradually increased to build up tolerance. AI #3 Capsule can be used to make the reaction less strong. After the reaction period is over, the patient should experience steady symptomatic improvement.

Symptoms similar to the Herxheimer's reaction may occur on a monthly basis for some patients. Generally speaking, a stronger Herxheimer's reaction may indicate a higher pathogen load in the body; consequently, treatment may need to be extended. The disappearance of these periodical symptom flare-ups can be used to determine the endpoint of treatment.

IV-7. Flowchart of MCM Herbal Treatments for Lyme Disease

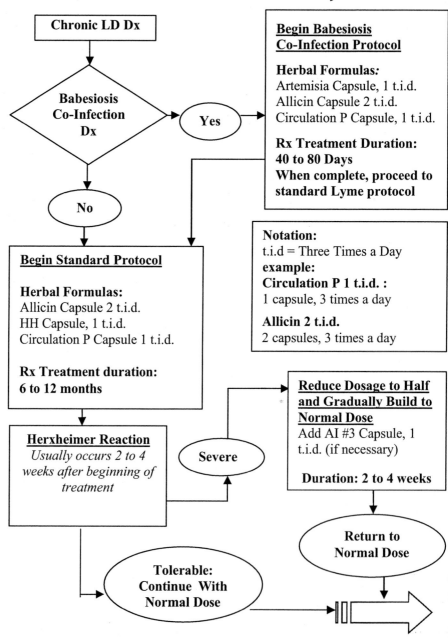

Chronic LD Dx

Babesiosis Co-Infection Dx

Yes

No

Begin Babesiosis Co-Infection Protocol

Herbal Formulas:
Artemisia Capsule, 1 t.i.d.
Allicin Capsule 2 t.i.d.
Circulation P Capsule, 1 t.i.d.

Rx Treatment Duration: 40 to 80 Days
When complete, proceed to standard Lyme protocol

Notation:
t.i.d = Three Times a Day
example:
Circulation P 1 t.i.d. :
1 capsule, 3 times a day

Allicin 2 t.i.d.
2 capsules, 3 times a day

Begin Standard Protocol

Herbal Formulas:
Allicin Capsule 2 t.i.d.
HH Capsule, 1 t.i.d.
Circulation P Capsule 1 t.i.d.

Rx Treatment duration: 6 to 12 months

Herxheimer Reaction
Usually occurs 2 to 4 weeks after beginning of treatment

Severe

Reduce Dosage to Half and Gradually Build to Normal Dose
Add AI #3 Capsule, 1 t.i.d. (if necessary)

Duration: 2 to 4 weeks

Return to Normal Dose

Tolerable: Continue With Normal Dose

<u>Continue Normal Dose Standard Protocol:</u>
<u>Add Individualized Formulas for Peripheral Conditions if Neccessary</u>

Allicin Odor Too Strong - Use Chlorophyll to reduce odor
(found at most health food stores)

Severe Fatigue: Add Cordyceps Capsule: 2 t.i.d.

Vasculitis, Fibromyalgia, MS-like symptoms, etc. -
Add AI #3: 2 capsules in the morning, 1capsule in the afternoon,
2 capsules in the evening (5 total per day)
Duration: 1 to 3 months, then discontinue

**Cognition problems, Memory loss, Mental fogginess, Concentration
problems:** Add Puerarin Capsule: 2 t.i.d.

Lyme Related Joint Pains and Arthritic Symptoms
Add Arthral EZ Tablet: 1 *t.i.d*

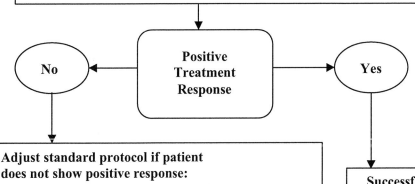

Positive Treatment Response

No

Yes

**Adjust standard protocol if patient
does not show positive response:**

Second-Line Protocol
Coptis Capsule (2 t.i.d.) or R-5081 Formula Capsule (2
t.i.d.) to replace Allicin Capsule.
Continue HH Capsule 1 t.i.d., Circulation P Capsule OR
(based on practitioner, Apply ABX treatment
concurrently)
Coptis Capsule 2 t.i.d. R-5081 Formula Capsule 2
t.i.d.Circulation P 1 t.i.d.

**Successfully
Complete
Standard
Treatment
Protocol**

Chapter V

Acupuncture for Lyme Disease

Since people know that acupuncture is effective for alleviating pain, many patients initially come to see us for arthritis pain. In many instances, we find that their pain could only be released by treating the underlying LD. Moreover, muscular-skeletal pain, such as arthritis and fibromyalgia, is a common LD symptom. Therefore, as an effective pain-releasing and immune- and circulation-regulating treatment, acupuncture plays an important role in treating LD.

According to the Gate Theory, the pain signal is carried by nerve fiber C at a speed of 10 meters per second, whereas the signal of acupuncture stimulation is carried by thicker A and B fibers at a speed of 100 meters per second. When the faster acupuncture signal arrives at the spinal neuron and excites it, the pain signal to the brain is interrupted. This mechanism explains the immediate effect of acupuncture.

The lasting effects of acupuncture are explained with the chemical endorphin theory. Acupuncture stimulation can cause the brain to secrete endorphin, a morphine-like pain-killer and a CNS immune regulator. In short, acupuncture releases the pain, while regulating immunity.

The brain images seen in functional magnetic resonance imaging (fMRI) have provided visual proof of acupuncture's pain-releasing effects. A study reported at the 85th Scientific Assembly and Annual Meeting of the Radiological Society of North America held in December 1999 showed markedly decreased brain activity triggered by pain in 57% of patients receiving manual acupuncture and 100% of patients receiving electro-acupuncture. The numbers corresponded to self-reported decreased levels of pain in the subjects. [39a]

Other new techniques, such as positron emission computerized tomography (PET) scan and SPECT scan, give an image of brain functions, such as how the brain utilizes glucose, its only energy source. These scans have shown that, when stroke patients undergo acupuncture treatments, some of their lost brain function is restored. [40,41] Because LD causes brain damage and since CNS symptoms are the major problem in chronic LD, acupuncture to restore brain function is an important LD treatment.

We use acupuncture points at the far extremities, such as *ba feng* points on the feet and *ba xie* points on the hands, which have strong effects on treating CNS symptoms. *He gu* (Li 4) and *tai chong* (Liv 3) are often used because they produce the strongest stimulation.

The recently developed scalp acupuncture has a very specific effect on the CNS symptoms and disorders. Scalp acupuncture also called cranial acupuncture or cephalic acupuncture. In 1989 the World Health Organization adopted the International Standard Nomenclature of Acupuncture and Moxibustion including Standard Nomenclature of Scalp Acupuncture points. Because this is a special technique in acupuncture, to consult a scalp acupuncture specialist is advised.

For joint pain and arthritis, we use points surrounding the joints, such as *qu chi* (Li 11) and *shou san li* (Li 10) for elbows; *ying ling quan* (Sp 9), *zu san li* (S 36), and *yang lin quan* (G 34) for knees; *jie xi* (S 41) for ankles; *pi guan* (S31) and *zu wu li* (Li 10) for hips; *jian yu* (Li 15), *nao shu* (Si 10), *jian zhen* (Si 9), and *tian liao* (Te 15) for shoulders; *wai guan* (Te 5) and *yang xi* (Li 5) for wrists.

We use acupuncture as an adjunctive treatment for LD, usually once or twice a week.

References for Chapter I to V

1. Burgdorfer W., et al., Lyme Disease – a tick borne spirochetosis? Science, 1982;216:1317

2. Ma Jin, The Research Progress in Pathogen of Lyme Disease, Chinese Journal of common disease of human and animal, 1989, 5:46

3. Cryan B., et al., Antimicrobial agent in Lyme disease, J Antimicrob Chemother, 1990, 25:187

4. Kenneth B. Liegner et al., Lyme disease and the Clinical Spectrum of Antibiotic Responsive Chronic Meningoencephalomyelitides, Proceedings of Lyme & Other Tick-borne Disease: A 21st Century View, Nov 10,2001, p.72

5. Nakata C et al., Analyt Biochem, 1970, 37:92

6. The Great Dictionary of Chinese Materia Medica, Shanghai Science and Technology Press, 1988, p.110-115

7. Ji YB, Pharmacological Action and Application of Available Composition of Traditional Chinese medicine, Helongjian Science and Technology Press, 1995, p.9

8. Yin Jian et al., The Modern Studies and Clinical Applications of Chinese Materia Medica, Volume 1, Xue Huan Press, 1994, p.86

9. Zhu Yan, Pharmacology and Applications of Chinese Materia Medica, People's Health Press, 1958, p.1

10. Wang Jiaying et al., Chinese Journal of Internal Medicine, (6): 549, 1959

11. Tang Pai, Chinese Journal of Medicine, 40(9): 721, 1954

12. The Chinese Medicine Research Group of Zhuong Qing Medical College, Journal of Microbiology (China), 8(1): 52, 1960

13. Dold H et al., C A, 47:9419, 1953

14. Yang SS, The Proceedings of First National Conference of Chinese Society of Physiology, 1956, p.26

15. Zao Renli et al., Chinese Journal of Dermatology, (4): 286, 1957

16. Zhang DJ et al., Chinese Journal of Medicine, 4(2): 126, 1957

17. Szynbna M et al., C A, 47, 2412, 1953

18. Yi HB et al., Acta Academica Medicina Primai Shanghai 1956 (1): 42

19. Chen XY, Chinese Journal of Abstracts and Gynecology 1956 (4): 395

20. Leptospirosis Research Unit, Chengdu College if traditional Chinese Medicine. Scientific Research Compilation. 3rd edition, Chengdu College of TCM, 1972. p.59

21. Yang HC et al., C A. 1953 47:8175d

22. Leptospirosis Research Unit, Sichuan Institute of Chinese Materia Medica. Research Information on TCM, 1971 (6):34

23. Jiangxi Medical Information (Jiangxi School of Pharmacy), 1972 (2):12

24. The Great Dictionary of Chinese Materia Medica, Shanghai Science and Technology Press,

    1988, p.91-93

25. Jaing et al., Foreign Medicine, Chinese Medicine, 1986, 8(2):54

26. Li et al., Trans Roy Soc Trop Med Hyg, 1983, 77(4):522

27. Qinghao Research Group, Journal of Traditional Chinese Medicine, 1982, 2(1):17

28. Yie ZG et al., Journal of Parasite and Parasitic Diseases, 1986, 4(4):260

29. Chen DJ et al., Chinese Medical Journal, 1980,60(7):422

29a. Zhuang GK., et al., New Medicine Journal, 1979; (6):39

30. Miyazake, et al., Chem Pharm Bull, 1977, (25):435

31. Liu RJ et al, Bulletin of Pharmaceutics, 1981, 16:567

32. Leptospirosis Research Unit, Chengdu College if traditional Chinese Medicine. Scientific Research Compilation. 3rd edition, Chengdu College of TCM, 1972. p.59

33. Yang HC et al., C A. 1953 47:8175d

34. Leptospirosis Research Unit, Sichuan Institute of Chinese Materia Medica. Research Information on TCM, 1971 (6):34

35. Jiangxi Medical Information (Jiangxi School of Pharmacy), 1972 (2):12

36. The Great Dictionary of Chinese Materia Medica, Shanghai Science and Technology Press, 1988, p.91-93

37. Jaing et al., Foreign Medicine, Chinese Medicine, 1986, 8(2):54

38. Li et al., Trans Roy Soc Trop Med Hyg, 1983, 77(4):522

39. Qinghao Research Group, Journal of Traditional Chinese Medicine, 1982, 2(1):17

39a. Anonymous, Brain images demonstrate that acupuncture relieves pain, Total Health; Jan/Feb 2000;22,1Research Library, p.12

40. Li Ji, et al., Influence of Acupuncture on Cerebral Glucose Metabolism in Patients with Cerebral Infarction, CJITWM, 2002, 22(10):741-744

41. Huang Y., et al., Effect of Scalp Acupuncture on Glucose Metabolism in Brain of Patients with Depression, CJITWM, 2005, 25(2):119-122

Chapter VI

Clinical Outcomes and Case Studies

Our clinic has treated more than 1,000 cases of LD, mostly in the chronic stages. Most patients have been able to taper off antibiotics and control their symptoms. After approximately six months or longer, the majority of them have completed herbal treatment and have remained symptom-free. MCM treatment for LD is designed to eradicate the pathogens; it is curative, not merely symptom-suppressing.

Determining a treatment endpoint is difficult, due to the lack of an accurate diagnostic test. Recently, with more accurate PCR tests to identify the existence of the pathogens, the majority of patients' PCR tests have turned negative following the MCM treatment course.

The cost of MCM herbal treatments is far less than the cost of conventional LD treatment. In "Lyme Disease: Cost to Society," published in the actuarial journal Contingencies, the average cost of treating LD through WM was found to be about $62,000 per patient. For MCM herbal treatments, the average cost is about $2,000 to $3,000. Besides, MCM treatments have far fewer and far less side effects, resulting in far less physical and mental stress for the patient. Unfortunately, herbal treatment is not covered by insurance, so the patient must bear the full cost.

Following are a few examples of the positive clinical results we have seen. They represent typical patients and typical outcomes. Their names were changed, but their stories are true.

VI-1: Case No. 1

Mr. L, a Pennsylvania computer consultant, was 39 when he came to our clinic for an initial visit on May 23, 1997, for his chronic LD, which had been diagnosed in October 1995. He had been suffering from neurological symptoms, fibromyalgia, Raynaud's syndrome, fatigue, food allergies, nausea, and irritable bowel syndrome for more than two years. He had been on and off antibiotics for more than a year, and during the three months prior to his initial visit had been on intravenous Rocephin. The prolonged antibiotics treatment had caused urinary-tract yeast infections, resulting in frequent, painful urination. He was very weak and fatigued. These symptoms prevented him from working regular hours. Despite the long-term intensive antibiotics treatment, he had seen little improvement with WM. Indeed, whenever he would discontinue antibiotics, his symptoms would return within a week or two. Yet, because antibiotics caused iatrogenic problems—urinary-tract infections, low white blood cell count, and irritable bowel syndrome—he felt that continued antibiotics treatment was not a viable option. As a result, he was prompted to come to our office.

He started the herbal treatment with Allicin Capsule, R-5081, Circulation P Capsule, and AI #3, as well as weekly acupuncture sessions. The first week he had very strong "die-off" symptoms (Herxheimer's reaction), and he reported increased mental fog. During the second week, however, he felt obvious improvement in his mental clarity. When he came for the third acupuncture treatment, which was also the third week of herbal treatment, he said that though this was his longest interval without antibiotics, his symptoms were improving. Nonetheless, he still reported body ache, fatigue, and numerous food allergies.

On June 21, 1997—the fourth week and still not using any antibiotics—his complexion evidenced much improvement. The grayish skin tone color was gone. He reported no cold hands or feet—the first time in years. He had more energy, had gained some weight, and was able to concentrate. He still, however, had body aches and back pain. Cordyceps Capsule was added to his protocol to enhance cellular immunity and to accelerate recovery. During the next three months, the problems caused by antibiotics—urinary-track infection, low WBC count, and irritable bowel syndrome—all gone. His entire course of treatment lasted seven months at our clinic, after which time he was able to return to work and resume his normal activities.

This case shows that long-term use of antibiotics causes iatrogenic problems. We have also seen patients who have been on long-term antibiotics exhibit highly elevated liver enzymes, gall bladder stones, and kidney damage. Herbal treatments have dramatically changed their prognosis.

VI-2: Case No. 2

Mr. N, 49, was diagnosed with both chronic LD and hepatitis C. He lives in British Columbia and so did not visit our New York clinic. Rather, all communication was handled by phone. He had been sick for more than a decade when he first contacted us on March 6, 2000. Unable to work or even walk or write, he had LD-induced motor nerve disease, which had resulted in loss of muscle strength, coordination, and balance. His dominant right side was semi-paralyzed; his right hand could not even reach his pocket. He also had cognitive problems, mental fog, arthritis, fibromyalgia, and swelling of the right knee joint. His WBC count was elevated and RBC was low. He had not been tested for babesiosis.

He had been diagnosed with hepatitis C by qualitative HCV RNA PCR test; the genotype of the virus was 1b. His circulating immune complexes test, RAJI cell- CIC, was off the scale, explaining the autoimmune symptoms of rheumatoid arthritis and fibromyalgia. Liver function tests showed that his enzymes were within the normal range, his liver disease was mild, and inflammation was dormant. He did not want to continue long-term antibiotics use because the hepatitis, though he used them short term with no improvement. Then he used colloidal silver, but he had concerns about heavy metal accumulation.

He began our herbal treatment mid-March 2000 with Artemisia Capsule, Allicin Capsule, AI #3 Capsule, and Circulation P Capsule. He had Herxheimer's reaction at first, but then reported steady, slow improvement. During the third month of treatment, we discontinued use of Artemisia Capsule and began use of HH Capsule, since during the first two months; the former was mainly for treating babesiosis.

His recovery took quite a long time because of his long infection history and the presence of hepatitis C. After his LD symptoms greatly improved, we started hepatitis C herbal treatment together with his LD treatment. Because LD herbs are virtually non-toxic and do not harm the liver, these two diseases can be treated simultaneously without treatments being at cross-purposes with each other. Circulation P Capsule was used to treat both diseases. After about two years of herbal treatment, Mr. N went back to work.

On Feb. 28, 2002, he wrote in perfectly legible handwriting: "Dr. Zhang, ... Have been back working just about full-time. Mercury detox is going well. What a confusing health challenge I have. Hope you and yours are well. Thank you."

Upon discontinuation of herbal treatment, Mr. N remained well, with only mild hepatitis C symptoms.

This case shows that herbal treatment is beneficial in patients with diseases for which conventional WM treatments may be at cross-purposes. Hepatitis C patients cannot tolerate long-term antibiotics, while LD patients have difficulty with interferon-based hepatitis C treatments. Our herbal protocols coordinate treatment of these two diseases, as well as the treatment of LD patients who also have inflammatory bowel disease.

VI-3: Case No. 3

Ms. S, 31, a teacher, came to our clinic on February 8, 2002, having been diagnosed with LD on October 1, 2001. Although she does not remember any tick bite or large skin rashes, she felt her symptoms had been present for three to 10 years. She reported mental fog, difficulty concentrating, exhaustion, multiple joint pain, body ache, hair loss, hypersensitivity to light, night sweats, pre-menstrual tension (PMS), and low libido. She also had multiple allergies to mold, dust, pollen, grass, trees, and animal hair. About 10 years before, she had suffered chronic fatigue syndrome. Because of arthritis-like symptoms, she visited a rheumatologist and tested ANA (+), as well as positive for LD. She completed six weeks of Doxycycline treatment, beginning in November 2001 and finishing on January 3, 2002, with no improvement. She then began looking for alternative treatment and found our clinic.

Her herbal treatment consisted of two months of Artemisia Capsule for babesiosis and Allicin Capsule and HH Capsule for treating *Bb* and other possible co-infections. Simultaneously, she used the TCM formula Tang-kuei and Evodia Combination for her PMS, as well as AI #3 and Circulation P to alleviate joint pain, suppress autoimmunity, and remove CIC. She also underwent weekly acupuncture treatment. Her PMS stopped after three months on the herbs. Her ANA turned to negative during the fourth month of treatment. The next month, she reported that most of her symptoms were gone. During the seventh month, PCR tests for *Bb* and babesiosis were negative. Her next five PCR tests all came back negative.

As is the case with most diseases, younger patients such as Ms. S generally respond better to treatment than do older patients. We have treated many LD patients in their 20s and 30s, and similar positive outcomes have been seen.

VI-4: Case No. 4

Ms. G, 55, a recreational therapist, visited our office on June 7, 1996, having been diagnosed with LD in 1993. Her main complaints were migraine headache, fatigue, and joint and muscle pain. She had been on and off antibiotics and anti-inflammatory medications since 1993. Her symptoms periodically flared up. Long-term use of antibiotics caused yeast infections, and she had developed a dependency on the anti-fungal drug Diaflucane to control these infections. She experienced a migraine almost every day. She had multiple allergies to pollen, dust, mold, wheat, and animals. She was one of our first LD patients, and at that time our LD treatment protocols were still being developed.

The main herbal remedy she used was a very purified, potent allicin solution, every vial of which contained 2ml of the solution with 30mg of *allitridi*. It had been developed in China for intravenous infusions. In the United States, it is used as a food supplement and it was administrated as a drink. Every vial of the solution dissolved in 8 ounces of water to be ingested twice a day. Because we found this substance so effective, we later developed a capsule form of allicin.

Ms. G also used an anti-syphilis formula mainly composed of Smilax glabra root, Baikal skullcap root (Scutellariae radix), and Chinese goldthread rhizome (Coptis chinensis Franch radix). From this early formulation, we developed the R-5081 Capsule. We used AI #3 to address her muscular-skeletal pain. Weekly acupuncture administered to her migraine and joint pain.

After seven months of treatment, most of her symptoms were gone. More than a decade ago—at the time of Ms. G's herbal treatment—few, if any, reliable laboratory tests were available. Moreover, babesiosis co-infection was not as common as it is now, so no anti-babesiosis treatment was undertaken. Our work with Ms. G helped us to develop more effective MCM treatments for our later LD patients.

Chapter VII
The Phytopharmacology of Herbal Remedies

MCM uses herbs according to both TCM principles and modern pharmacological studies. This chapter presents the phytopharmacology of the herbal remedies we developed for treating LD. Most of them have been used in our clinical practice for more than a decade. They are prime examples of the modernization of TCM herbal remedies. For every herbal formula, the constituent herbs, their botanical name, chemical components, pharmacological actions, clinical studies and applications in China, and packaging and dosage are provided.

Botanical names are necessary for plant identification. English common names cannot uniquely identify the correct species because many herbs have similar common names. Moreover, some species are indigenous to China and do not have English names.

Thanks to the TCM modernization movement, now we can use phytochemical studies of TCM herbs to recognize and isolate active ingredients and purify them. By using the purified active ingredients, we can avoid contaminations from chemical fertilizers, pesticides, and heavy metals. The potency and consistency of herbal formulas can also be accurately measured.

Phytopharmacological studies on these active ingredients were conducted on animal models, in cell cultures, and in microbial cultures. These studies explored and specified the physiological and microbiological effects of the herb and/or its constituents. Because the herbs have already been in TCM clinical use, their therapeutic effects are either confirmed by the tests or the effects can be used to explain the mechanism of the therapeutic actions. From these studies, the toxicity indicator, $LD_{50,}$ and the efficacy indicator, ED_{50}, were also determined. From these, the therapeutic safety index, $LD_{50}/ED_{50,}$ was calculated—an important factor in the safe application of the herb.

The clinical studies done in China have given us practical guidance on how to apply these herbs in our own clinic. Some treatments can be "borrowed" from herb protocols used for similar diseases. For example, herbs effective in treating syphilis and leptospirosis have shown to be effective against similar microbial infections such as LD. Our work is focused on how to match the pathogenesis of LD with similar diseases and corresponding treatments. For more than 10 years, we have been studying and treating LD. Our treatment has matured, but we continue to improve our protocol.

These herbal products were produced under the Good Manufacture Practice (GMP) standards. For them to be exported from China and imported to the United States, they must meet strict criteria. They have to pass residual tests for heavy metals, bacteria, and chemicals. Because they were designed by us and produced under our supervision, we are confident of their potency and high quality.

VII-1: Herbal Remedies Developed by and Used in the Zhang Clinic

Herbal Formula Intake Guide	
AI #3 Capsule	One capsule three times a day with meals; or for higher dosage, two in the morning, one at noon, and two in the evening.
	Caution: This capsule should only be used for reducing the severity of Herxheimer's reaction, or for joint pain, skin rash, autoimmune reactions, and allergies. It should be stopped after these symptoms are no longer present. The treatment course with this herbal remedy should be limited to three months. If treatment must be resumed, wait at least one month before resuming use.

Allicin Capsule	Two to three capsules (dependent on body weight, 2mg of allitridi/kg/day) three times a day, with meals.
Artemisia Capsule	One capsule three times a day before meals.
ArthralEZ Tablet	One tablet three times a day with meals.
Circulation P Capsule	One capsules three times a day before meals.
Coptis Capsule	Two capsules three times a day before meals.
Cordyceps Capsule	Two capsules three times a day before meals.
R-5081 Capsule	One capsules three times a day before meals.
HerbSom Capsule	Two capsules at bedtime.
HH Capsule	One capsule three times a day before meals.
Puerarin Capsule	Two capsules three times a day before meals.

VII-2: AI #3 Capsule

Constituent Herbs

Mucunae caulis, Sargentodoxae caulis, and *Paederiae caulis*

Pharmacology

Mucunae caulis, botanical name is *Spatholobus suberectus* Dunn. In TCM it is considered bittersweet and warm-propertied. It is used for promoting blood circulation and treating irregular menstruation and weak legs.[1] Pharmacological studies found that it can noticeably suppress arthritis caused by formaldehyde in rat models. It has sedative and sleep-inducing effects. Clinically, it has been used for amenorrhea and leukemia caused by radiation. [2]

Sargentodoxae caulis, botanical name is *Sargentodoxa cuncata* (Oliv.) Rehd et Wils. Bitter and mild, according to TCM, it reduces swelling, promotes blood circulation, and activates collateral flow. Clinically, it is used for treating acute and chronic appendicitis, irregular menstruation, and rheumatism. Pharmacological studies found it can suppress various bacteria, such as *Staphylococcus aureus, Streptococcus,* and *Pseudomonas aeruginosa.* In modern clinical applications, it has been used to treat leprosy, rheumatic arthritis, and appendicitis. [3]

Paederiae caulis, botanical name is *Paederia scandens* (Lour.) Merr. Mild-propertied and sweet with a slightly bitter aftertaste, it is anti-rheumatic, anti-tussive, mucolytic, and analgesic. It is used to treat rheumatic pain, injuries due to impact, fractures, contusions and strains, eczema, and skin ulcers.

Pharmacological studies found that it has analgesic and sedative actions. It can raise the pain threshold and prolong pentobarbital sodium-induced sleep. The total alkaloids of this herb inhibited the contraction of the isolated intestine and antagonized spasm due to acetylcholine and histamine. It has expectorant, antibacterial, hypotensive, and local anesthetic actions. It has a high LD_{50} and has virtually no toxicity. Clinically, it has been used for many skin diseases, such as eczema, neurodermatitis, lepromatous leprosy, and respiratory tract diseases, such as bronchitis and whooping cough. It has corticoid-cortisone like effects. [4]

Clinical Applications

*Autoimmune disorders, such as rheumatoid arthritis, psoriasis, inflammatory bowel diseases, and systematic lupus erythematosus

* Allergic reactions and skin rashes
* Herxheimer's reaction, fibromyalgia, and joint pain

Packaging and Dosage

Each capsule contains 100mg of the extracts of the formula.

One bottle contains 50 capsules. Take one capsule, three times a day, or follow healthcare provider's advice.

Caution

This formula has humeral-immunity suppressive effects; only use when needed. It should be stopped after three months of continuous use for an interval of one month before resuming intake to avoid immune suppression. It may cause menstrual irregularities in women of childbearing age. If so, use should be limited to three months. Menstrual changes are reversible.

References

1. The Great Dictionary of Chinese Materia Medica, Shanghai Science and Technology Press, 1988, p.1206-1207
2. Xu J et al., Pharmacology and Clinics of Chinese Materia Medica, 1993, 9(4): 30
3. The Great Dictionary of Chinese Materia Medica, Shanghai Science and Technology Press, 1988, p.122-123
4. The Great Dictionary of Chinese Materia Medica, Shanghai Science and Technology Press, 1988, p.1214-1215

VII-3: Allicin Capsule

Constituent Herb

Allium sativa (garlic)

Garlic has a long history of medical applications. TCM describes it as warm-propertied with an acrid taste. Traditionally, it is used as a *qi* (vital energy) stimulant. It has stomach-warming, digestant, anti-inflammatory, detoxifying, and anti-helminthes effects. It is used for indigestion, diarrhea, dysentery, whooping cough, carbuncle, furuncle, tinea capitis, edema, snakebites, and insect stings. [1]

Chemical Composition

Highly purified and concentrated garlic essence: *allitridi*.

Its chemical name is diallyl thiosulfonate (2-propene-1-sulfinothioic acid, S-2-propenyl ester).

Its molecular structure is $CH_2=CHCH_2-S=O-SCH_2CH=CH_2$.

Its molecular formula is $C_6H_{10}OS_2$ and molecular weight is 162.27 daltons. [2]

Garlic bulb contains volatile oil, of which alliin is the major constituent. When the fresh bulb is macerated, alliin is decomposed into allicin by allinase. The characteristic odor of garlic is due to allicin. In the market today you can buy many kinds of deodorized garlic products, which are not useful for anti-infection, since the garlic odor carries the anti-infection properties. [3]

Allicin Capsule is made in a time-released form, thereby ensuring even dispersal.

Pharmacology

1. Anti-microbial effects

Pharmacological studies found that it has a very wide anti-microbial spectrum, with anti-bacterial, anti-mycobacterium, anti-fungal, anti-protozoal, and anti-viral properties.

a. Anti-bacterial effects

A 0.5% aqueous solution of the bulb was lethal to *Salmonella typhi* within five minutes of contact. It was significantly bacteriostatic or bactericidal against the following: *Staphylococci, Neisseria meningitides, Streptococcus pneumonia, Shigelia dysentery, Corynebacterium diphtheriae, Escherichia coli, Salmonella typhi* and *paratyphi, Mycobacterium tuberculosis, var. hominis,* and *Vibrio cholerae.* Bacteria resistant to penicillin, streptomycin, chloramphenicol, and chlortetracycline were sensitive to *allitridi,* the highly purified chemical precursor of allicin. The mechanism of the anti-bacterial action of allitridi involved a combination of its oxygen atom with cysteine to avert the formation of cystine, thus interrupting essential oxidation and reduction reactions in the bacteria. [4,5,6,7,8]

b. Anti-fungal effects

Anti-fungal action was observed *in vitro* against *Schlemm's Dermatomyces flavosa, Trichophyton vilaceum*, and *Candida albicans. In vitro* tests proved that 1-1.25 mcg/ml of diallyl thiosulfonate was inhibitory against *Candida albicans*, as was 0.05-1 mcg/ml to *Cryptococcus rubrae* and 3.2-12.5 mcg/ml to *Cryptococcus*. The minimum inhibitory dose of *allitridi* on fungi was 1mcg/ml; its effect was about the same as that of amphotericin B, but was far less toxic for test subjects. [9,10,11,12]

c. Anti-protozoal effects

The ameba *trophozoites* soon lost activity upon direct contact with the 5-15% aqueous suspension of the bulb. Experiments using direct contact and fumigation methods showed that garlic juice killed all *Trichomonas* organisms in 10-25 minutes, and the volatile components in 90-180 minutes, whereas 0.5% of the bulb filtrate deactivated *Trichomonas vaginalis* in five minutes. A 0.1% injective preparation of the bulb was lethal to tsutsugarnushi fever, including richettsiasis. [4,13,14]

2. Anti-neoplastic and other effects

Allitridi has anti-neoplastic (tumor) effects. It has anti-mitotic action against the cells of ascites sarcoma

MTK-1 in rats and those of Ehrlich ascites carcinoma in mice. [15,16] The fresh garlic bulb fed to C_3H/He female mice completely suppressed breast cancer. The active component might be allicin. [17] In ascitic and solid types of liver carcinoma in mice, garlic oil significantly prolonged the survival period of the animals. Marked inhibitory action was detected against many solid sarcoma in animals after intraperitoneal or intra-tumor injection of the oil at a dose of 50-100 mg/kg; the inhibition rate was 40-50%. [18] The anti-mitotic effect of the synthetic garlic oil on cancer cells, which eventually led to cell death, was more pronounced and stable than that of the natural garlic oil. The main anti-neoplastic component is diallyl thiosulfonate (*allitridi*). [19] This garlic ingredient also has immune-enhancing [20] and blood lipid-reducing effects. [21, 22]

3. Pharmacokinetics

After intake of S^{35}-labeled *allitridi* orally, the total radioactivity in organs peaked in four hours, and in eight hours it was reduced to half of the peak value. After intravenous injection of *allitridi* into mice, concentrations detected 10 minutes later were highest in the lungs, and in descending order in the heart, intestines, blood, fat, brain, muscles, spleen, and liver. The metabolism of *allitridi* in the body was very rapid; most of the intravenous dose was transformed into water-soluble metabolites within 10 minutes and was rapidly distributed to all organs. The main route of excretion was the urine, and, secondarily, the feces. [19, 23, 24]

4. Toxicity

It has almost no toxicity, with an LD_{50} of 134.9mg/kg in mice at 67.45-134.9 times higher its therapeutic dose (1-2 mg/kg). [19] Rabbits fed with 0.15% of *allitridi* at a dose of 3ml/kg twice daily for 10 weeks showed no pathological changes in the liver, spleen, adrenal glands, and lungs. *Allitridi* is a very safe substance. [25]

Clinical Applications [4,26,27,28]

❖ Lyme Disease, as an anti-spirochete agent, because it easily passes the blood brain barrier and so is especially beneficial in treating CNS infections

❖ Bacterial infections, especially bronchitis, sinusitis, and tuberculosis, especially drug-resistant TB

❖ Fungal infections, especially candidiasis and deep fungal infections

❖ Protozoa infections, especially amebic dysentery

Allitirdi has been clinically used in China for more than 20 years. It is potent enough to treat many common infections, such as bacillary dysentery, amebic dysentery, deep fungal infections (cryptococcus maligitis), whooping cough, endobronchial tuberculosis, toxoplasmosis, oxyuriasis, and trichomonas vaginitis. For most of these conditions, the cure rate is above 80%. Recent studies done by the AIDS Research Alliance in Los Angeles, as well as our clinical work, have found that it can be used to treat cryptosporidiosis. [29] Our clinic has been using this substance successfully to treat many infectious conditions.

Packaging and Dosage

Every bottle contains 30 or 60 capsules. Every capsule contains 20mg of *allitridi*. For prevention, take one capsule per day. For infections, take two to three capsules, three times a day with food.

References

1. The Great Dictionary of Chinese Materia Medica, Shanghai Science and Technology Press, 1988, p.110-115

2. Ji YB, Pharmacological Action and Application of Available Composition of Traditional Chinese medicine, Helongjian Science and Technology Press, 1995, p.9

3. Yin Jian et al., The Modern Studies and Clinical Applications of Chinese Materia Medica, Volume 1, Xue Huan Press, 1994, p.86

4. Zhu Yan, Pharmacology and Applications of Chinese Materia Medica, People's Health Press, 1958, p.1

5. Wang Jiaying et al., Chinese Journal of Internal Medicine, (6): 549, 1959

6. Tang Pai, Chinese Journal of Medicine, 40(9): 721, 1954

7. The Chinese Medicine Research Group of Zhuong Qing Medical College, Journal of Microbiology (China), 8(1): 52, 1960

8. Dold H et al., C A, 47:9419, 1953

9. Yang SS, The Proceedings of First National Conference of Chinese Society of Physiology, 1956, p.26

10. Zao Renli et al., Chinese Journal of Dermatology, (4): 286, 1957

11. Zhang DJ et al., Chinese Journal of Medicine, 4(2): 126, 1957

12. Szynbna M et al., C A, 47, 2412, 1953

13. Yi HB et al., Acta Academica Medicina Primai Shanghai 1956(1): 42

14. Chen XY, Chinese Journal of Abstracts and Gynecology 1956(4): 395

15. Kimura Y et al., C A 1966 63:1089d

16. Kroening K et al., C A 1964 61:15206c

17. Tumor Prevention and Treatment Group, 184 Hospital of Chinese PLA, Proceedings of the National Conference on Cooperative Research on Anti-Cancer Drugs, 1978, p.15

18. Pharmacology Department, Hunan Medical College, Proceedings of the National Conference on Cooperative Research on Anti-Cancer Drugs, 1978, p.1

19. Cytology Research Group of Tumor Research Unit of Hunan Medical College, Special Edition of National Conference on Cooperative Research on Anti-Cancer Drugs, 1977

20. TCM Department, First Teaching Hospital of Hunan Medical College, Chinese Traditional and Herbal Drugs Communication 1976 (12): 29

21. Qian BC, Academy of TCM, The References of TCM Review, 1979 (1): 40

22. Bordia A et al., Arteriosclerosis, 1975 21(1): 15

23. Fortunatov MN, Farmakologiia I Toksilologia (Russian) 1955 18(4): 43

24. Shanghai No.2 Pharmaceutical Factory, Abstracts of Research Information on 35S-Allicin as Tracer in Mice. April 1979

25. Shanghai No.2 Pharmaceutical Factory, Chinese Traditional and Herbal Drugs Communication 1976 (10): 8

26. Ren CO et al., Northeastern Region Medical Journal 1952 (7): 617

27. Third People's Hospital, Shanghai Second Medical College, Chinese Traditional and Herbal Drugs Communication 1973 (2): 53

28. TCM Department, First Teaching Hospital of Shanghai Second Medical College, Medical Research Communication 1977 (6): 39

29. Fareed, G et al., First Study of high-dose Garlic Preparation Shows Promise for the Treatment of Cryptosporidum parvum Diarrhea. Searchlight, Spring, 1996, p.16

VII-4: Artemisia Capsule

Constituent Herbs

Main herb: *Artemiciae apiacea* Hance or *Artemisiae annua* L. Auxillary herbs: *Astragalus membranaceus* and *Codonopsis pilosula*. The following discussion pertains only to the main herb, artemisia. [1]

Chemical Composition

Chinese name: *qing hao su*[2]

Chemical name: 3,13 – epoxy – 12H – pyrano [4,3-j] – 1,2-benzodioxepin –10(3H) one, cctahydro –3,6,9 – trimethyl -, [3R –(3 ,5 , 6 , 8 , 9 , 12 , 12 R)]-.

Molecular formula: $C_{15}H_{22}O_5$

Molecular weight: 282.14 [3,4]

Pharmacology

- ❖ Anti-malarial effects: Pharmacological studies found *qing hao su* (arteannuin or Artemisinin) and its derivative artesunate has strong anti-malarial action. Arteannuin and artesunate were lethal to *Endoerythrocytic plasmodium*. Symptomatic control and negative *plasmodium* examination were achieved rapidly by using them compared with chloroquine. Resistance of *plasmodia* to arteannuin developed at a much slower rate than to chloroquine. Arteannuin is effective against chloroquine-resistant strains. The drawback is its high relapse rate. Improvement in the molecular structure of the active ingredient has reduced relapse rate, such as artesunate, especially when it was used with *Astragalus membranaceus* and *Codonopsis pilosula*. [4,5,6,7,8,9] Pharmacological studies also found that paraaminobezoic acid or folic acid did not antagonize its anti-malarial action. There was no synergistic action between this agent and sulfamethozine. Therefore, its anti-malarial action was probably unrelated to folic-acid metabolism. It was shown that when arteannuin was used with trimethoprim in rat malaria, its anti-malarial action was enhanced and the relapse rate following discontinuation of the agent was also decreased. *In vitro* culture indicated that arteannuin has a direct lethal effect on *plasmodium*.

❖ Under the electron microscope, it was found that the site of its action was on the membranous structures of the endoerythrocytic asexual *plasmodium*, primarily on the food vacuole membrane, surface membrane, and mitochondrial membrane, and secondarily on the nuclear membrane and endoplasmic reticulum. It also affected the intra-nuclear chromosomes. The alteration of the food vacuole membrane interrupted the nutrition intake of the *plasmodium*. Following the deprivation of amino acids, auto-phagocytic vacuoles were found that were continually excreted out of the protozoa, resulting in the loss of large amounts of cytoplasm, destruction of the internal structure, and death of the parasites.[10,11,12,13,14]

❖ Anti-*Babesia* effects: The use of *qing hao su* in treating babesiosis was a "hunch" by the author, based on the similarity of babesiosis and malaria, and the fact that conventional WM uses anti-malarial therapies to treat babesiosis. We have had good success in using arteannuin to treat babesiosis. Moreover, compared with WM treatment, it has shown far fewer side effects and requires a shorter therapeutic course.

❖ Anti-schistosomiasis effects [15,16]

❖ Cardiovascular effects, specifically, heart-rate reduction, blood-pressure reduction, and arrhythmia alleviation. [17]

❖ Immune-regulatory effects: Serum interferon level increased and maintained at the elevated level for 24 hours in mice who were given *qing hao su*. Increased phagocytic activity started 24 hours after administration and stayed elevated for 72 hours. It increased the percentage of phagocytosis of phagocytes up to 53.1% and increased phagocytic index to 1.91. The elevated phagocytic activity may be a result of the effects of interferon. It can reduce serum IgG in sensitized animals and increase the weight of the spleen. It has obvious suppressive effects on humeral and cellular immunity. In mice, its administration can reduce the amount of antibody production cells and also suppress delayed allergic reactions, as well as suppress IL-2 production in mice spleen. These effects explain its usage in treating systematic lupus erythematosus. [18,19,20,21,22]

❖ Anti-cancer effects, specifically the promotion of apoptosis of cancerous cells.

Toxicity

Studies have found that *qing hao su* is widely dispersed and rapidly absorbed, metabolized, and excreted. There was no accumulation after long-term use of this substance. [23,24,25,26,27]

Its LD_{50} for intramuscular, intraceliac, and subcutaneous injection were 2,800, 1,558, and 9,000 mg/kg, respectively. Its therapeutic index was 36.80, compared to chloroquine's of 28.8, making it safer than chloroquine. The herb *qing hao* and its essence arteannuin are very low in toxicity. [17,28,29]

Clinical Applications

❖ Malaria: A 100% cure rate was achieved in 485 cases of tertian malaria and 105 cases of subtertian malaria. These two groups were all treated with a tablet made from the dilute alcohol extract of the herb at a total dose of 86.4g of crude herb in divided doses over three days. Arteannuin evidenced fast-acting anti-pyretic and anti-plamodial actions. [30]

❖ Babesiosis: In our clinic, one treatment course is generally 40 to 80 days. Most patients see their babesiosis test turn to negative after one course. Very few need a second course.

❖ SLE (systematic lupus erythematosus) and lupus erythematosus discoides: Almost every case experienced remission in varying degrees. At the beginning of treatment, however, symptoms may temporarily worsen. [31,32]

Packaging and Dosage

Each capsule contains 500mg of the extracts of *Artemisiae annua L. herba*, *Astragalus membranaceus*, and *Codonopsis pilosula*. Take one capsule, three times a day.

References

1. The Great Dictionary of Chinese Materia Medica, Shanghai Science and Technology Press, 1988, p.1228-1229
2. Ji YB, Pharmacological Action and Application of Available Composition of Traditional Chinese Medicine, Helongjian Science and Technology Press, 1994, p. 42-45

3. Qinghao Research Group, Science Bulletin (Chinese), 1977:22(3):142
4. Qinghao Research Group, Science Bulletin (Chinese), 1979:14(2):49
5. UNDP/World Bank/WHO. TDR/CHEMALSWG (4)/(QHS)/ 1981(3)
6. Jian QB et al., The lancet, 1982, 8(7):285
7. Guan WJ et al., Academe Journal of Second Military Medical University, 1986, 7(2):123
8. Xuan WJ et al., Academic Journal of Materia Medica (Chinese),1990, 25(3):220
9. Yie B et al., Academic Journal of Materia Medica (Chinese),1991, 26(3):228
10. Eillis et al., Ann Troo Med Parasito, 1985, 79(4):367
11. Jaing et al., Foreign Medicine, Chinese Medicine, 1986, 8(2):54
12. Li et al., Trans Roy Soc Trop Med Hyg, 1983, 77(4):522
13. Qinghao Research Group, Journal of Traditional Chinese Medicine, 1982, 2(1):17
14. Yie ZG et al., Journal of Parasite and Parasitic Diseases, 1986, 4(4):260
15. Chen DJ et al., Chinese Medical Journal, 1980,60(7):422
16. Lu WJ et al., Academic Journal of Materia Medica (Chinese),1981, 16(8):516
17. Li S et al., Journal of New Chinese Medicine, 1979 (6):51
18. Lin BY et al., Academic Journal of Materia Medica (Chinese),1985, 20(3):211
19. Shen M et al., Chinese Science B, 1983, 10:928

20. Zhang D et al., Chinese Pharmacology Bulletin, 1989, 5(1):37

21. Chen H et al., Academic Journal of Penbu Medical College, 1988, 13(3):195

22. Qien RS et al., Journal of Traditional Chinese Medicine, 1981, 6:63

23. Zhao KC et al., Academic Journal of Materia Medica (Chinese),1988, 21(10):736

24. Chen S et al., Journal of New Chinese Medicine, 1980 (1):37

25. Zhu DY et al., Academic Journal of Materia Medica (Chinese),1980, 15(8):509

26. Zhu DY et al., Chinese Academic Journal of Pharmacology, 1983, 4(3):194

27. Research Group on Qinghaosu and Its Derivatives as Antimalarials, J Trad Chin Med, 1982,2(1):25

28. Ning DX et al., Chin J of Pharmacology and Toxicology, 1987, 1(2):135

29. Institute of Pharmacology of Chinese Academe of TCM, Journal of New Medicine, 1979, (1):23

30. Fan TT et al., Journal of New Chinese Medicine, 1988, 20(1):35

31. Wang GY et al., Middle Rank Medical Journal 1981,(7):39

32. Zhuang GK et al., Journal of New Chinese Medicine, 1979 (6):39

VII-6: Arthral EZ Tablet

Arthritis and fibromyalgia (muscular pain), which affect tens of millions of people, are also major symptoms of Lyme disease and viral hepatitis. Besides treating the underlying disorders, we sought to alleviate the suffering of our patients in order to improve their quality of life. This is why we adopted this combination of Western and Chinese herbal dietary supplement as part of our protocol. It has both localized effects and systemic blood circulation-regulating actions to release muscular-skeletal pain.

Arthral EZ Tablet is a natural arthritis treatment specifically formulated with clinically proven ingredients that have been shown to safely reduce the pain and discomfort of common arthritis and address the symptoms of joint degeneration. No other natural arthritis treatment is as comprehensive, or as effective. Stephen Paul, Ph.D. of biochemistry, who is an authority in the dietary supplement industry, formulated Arthral EZ.

Within Arthral EZ, anti-inflammatory, analgesic, and rehabilitating ingredients create a powerful formula more effective than other brands or than any one ingredient by itself. This combination provides pain relief from arthritis without drugs like aspirin or ibuprofen. This means that the user will not suffer any of the associated side effects of pain-killers. Arthral EZ

Tablet is safe for people with ulcers, gastritis, hepatitis, and colitis.

Ingredients

Glucosamine, manganese ascorbate, chondroitin sulfate, Type II collagen, vitamin C, and the Chinese herbs *san qi* (*Panax notoginseng*), *dang gui* (*Angelicae sinensis radix*), *chuan xiong* (*Cnidii rhizoma*), *luo xin fu gen* (*Astilbes chinensis radix*), and *hong hua* (*Carthami flos*).

Pharmacology

❖ Glucosamine is a key component of cartilage and so works to stimulate joint function and repair. It has been proven effective in numerous scientific trials for treating osteo-arthritis pain, rehabilitating cartilage, renewing joint fluid, and repairing joints that have been damaged from osteo-arthritis.

❖ Manganese ascorbate enhances the beneficial effects of glucosamine sulfate and chondroitin in combating arthritis.

❖ Chondroitin sulfate, a normal component of joint cartilage, reduces destructive enzymes in the joints and increases constructive enzymes. It is as effective as NSAIDs for osteo-arthritis.

❖ Type II collagen has shown great efficacy in relieving joint pain, particularly in osteo-arthritis. It is one of the proteins that is under immune attack in rheumatoid arthritis. By taking Type II collagen, the immune system becomes tolerant to the Type II collagen in cartilage and stops attacking it.

❖ Vitamin C is essential for repair and maintenance of cartilage. It also acts as an antioxidant to offset the damage of free radicals.

❖ The Chinese herbs *san qi* (*Panax notoginseng*), *dang gui* (*Angelicae sinensis radix*), *chuan xiong* (*Cnidii rhizoma*), *luo xin fu gen* (*Astilbes chinensis radix*), and *hong hua* (*Carthami flos*) are formulated for their powerful blood circulation-promoting and stasis-expelling actions. According to TCM theory, pain is mainly caused by blood stasis. To release pain and aches, one must promote blood circulation and expel stasis. These five Chinese herbs also contain proven pain-killing effects and can improve overall health by improving blood circulation.

Clinical Applications

Arthral EZ Formula has been shown to help reduce joint and muscle pain and inflammation, reduce joint stiffness, restore healthy joint movement and range of motion, repair damaged cartilage in joints, maintain healthy joint fluid, and speed recovery of injured joints.

Packaging and Dosage

One bottle contains 90 tablets (one-month supply), with 1000mg per tablet. Take one tablet three times a day with meals.

VII-6: Circulation P Capsule

Constituent Herbs

Carthami flos, Persicae semen, Angelicae radix, Cnidii rhizoma, Rehmanniae radix, Paeoniae rubra radix, Achyranthis radix, Bupleuri radix, Glycyrrhizae radix, and *Platycodi radix.*

Traditional Use

Circulation P Capsule is a modification of the TCM formula Persica and Achyranthes Combination (*xue fu zhu yu tang*) and Persica and Cnidium Combination (*ge xia zhu yu tang*). Traditionally, these two formulas were used for blood stasis, typically with symptoms of dark or purplish tongue, cold hands and feet, dark rings around the eyes, liver palms, spider moles, dry and itchy skin, rashes, and upper abdominal discomfort. [1]

Pharmacology

❖ Improves microcirculation: This formula can noticeably ameliorate acute microcirculation disorders induced by macromolecular dextran in rats. It dilates micro-capillaries, accelerates blood flow, and opens more micro-capillary networks. The result is to increase blood infusion to the tissues and stop the pathology caused by the microcirculation disorder. [2] Additionally, it can clear the clotting factors in

DIC (diffuse intravenous coagulation) and stop the progress of DIC. It can suppress the clustering of platelets and improve blood liquidity, but will not prolong prothrombin time. [3]

❖ Enhances phagocytosis of the macrophages to remove CIC and regulates cellular and humeral immunity. [4]

❖ Noticeably suppresses granuloma formation. [5]

Clinical Applications

❖ Used in inflammatory diseases to promote healing of inflamed tissue, such as is seen in chronic gastritis, costal chondritis, and dermatitis. [6,7,8]

❖ Chronic hepatitis: It can promote the normalization of liver function, shrink an enlarged liver and spleen, promote the absorption of ascites, and improve overall blood circulation, though it should be used in conjunction with other liver-protecting herbs. [9]

❖ Cirrhosis: The Tianjing Institute of Emergent Medicine in Tianjing, China, used it to treat 18 cases of ascites caused by cirrhosis and found its effectiveness to be 94%. It helps to improve microcirculation in the liver. [10]

Besides the above-mentioned applications, it has been extensively used in internal medicine, gynecology, and surgery.

Packaging and Dosage

Each capsule contains 500mg of the herbal extracts of the formula. One bottle contains 45 capsules, enough for 15 days. Take one capsules three times a day before meals.

References

1. Bai G et al., Research and Applications of Chinese Herbal Formulas, Chinese Science and Technology Press, 1995, p.403 -411

2. Fang QL, Chinese Patent Medicine, 1988, (7):29

3. Tienjin First Center Hospital, Chinese J of Internal Medicine, 1977, 2(2):79

4. Zhang LR, Tienjin Medical J., 1987, 15 (9):544

5. Fong YJ, Shuanxi J of TCM, 1988, 9(3):126

6. Wu JL, Academic J of Henan College of TCM, 1978, (2):28

7. Zhang RJ, J TCM, 1980, 21 (6):35

8. Bien TJ, Chinese J of Dermatology, 1980, (1):57

9. Shi ZS, J of New Medicine, 1978, (9):36

10. Yang JY, J New Chinese medicine, 1987, 19(5):48

VII-7: Coptis Capsule

Constituent Herb

Coptis chinensis Franch, the major chemical ingredient of which is umbellatine. [1,2]

Pharmacology

❖ Anti-bacterial actions: Coptis can strongly suppress *Staphylococcus aureus, Streptococcu, pneumococcus, Vibrio comma, Anthrax bacillus,* and *Bacillus dysenteriae.* It can also suppress *Hay bacillus, Pneumobacillus, Bacillus diphtheriae, Bordetella pertussis, Brucellaceae,* and *Mycobacterium tuberculosis.* Its potency is roughly equal to or stronger than that of sulfanilamide and slightly weaker than that of streptomycin and chloramphenicol. It has strong bacteriocidal effects on spirochete. [3,4,5,6,7,8,9]

❖ Anti-viral actions: It has been shown to suppress influenza viruses and Newcastle disease virus in *in vitro* tests. [10,11,12,13]

❖ Anti-fungal, anti-amebic, and anti-*Chlamydi trachomatis,* -*trichomonad,* and -*Leptospira.* [14,15,16,17,18,19]

❖ Anti-neoplastic [20,21,22], anti-radiation[23,24,25], and blood sugar-regulating effects. [26] In treating chronic hepatitis, its bile-secretion-facilitating effect is especially useful. [27,28,29,30]

❖ Toxicity: It is a very safe herbal remedy, with virtually no side effects. Long-term use has not caused any adverse reactions and no accumulative toxicity. LD_{50} for rats is 205mg/kg [31,32,33].

Clinical Applications

❖ Coptis has a wide anti-infectious spectrum and has been used for treating bacterial infections such as abscess, bacillary dysentery, and gastritis. [34, 35]

❖ Chronic gall bladder inflammation, for which coptis has shown an efficacy rate of 88.2%. [36]

❖ Respiratory infections, such as bronchitis, sinusitis, and tonsillitis. [37]

❖ Protozoa infections, such as amebic dysentery, *trichomonas vaginitis*, and candidiasis. [38]

❖ Type II diabetes, cardiac arrhythmia, and hypertension. [38]

Packaging and Dosage

Every bottle contains 90 capsules. Take two capsules three times a day.

References

1. The Great Dictionary of Chinese Materia Medica, Shanghai Science and Technology Press, 1988, p.2022-2030

2. Ji YB, Pharmacological Action and Application of available composition of TCM, Helongjiang Science and Technology Press, 1994, p.69-70

3. Xu ZL, Chinese Medical Journal, 1947, 33:71

4. Chen MR, Acta Academiae Medicinae Sichuan (Special Edition on Comprehensive Studies of Coptis) 1955 (1):55

5. Xu ZL, Acta Academiae Medicinae Sichuan (Special Edition on Comprehensive Studies of Coptis) 1955 (1):41

6. Gao SY et al., Science 1949, 110(1):11

7. Liao YX, Acta Pharmaceutica Sinica, 1954, 2(1):5

8. Zhao CY et al., Acta Microbiologica Sinica 1960, (8):171

9. Amin AH et al., Canadian J of Microbiology, 1969,15:1067

10. Ye YL et al., Chinese Medical Journal, 1958, 44(9):888

11. Gao SY, Science Record 1950, 3(2-4):231

12. Zhang TM et al., Chinese Medical Journal, 1957, 43(8):627

13. Kulkarin SK et al., The Japanese J of Pharmacology 1972, 22(1):11

14. Sabit M et al., Indian J Med Research, 1976, 64(8):1160

15. Ob-Gyn Department, Bulletin of Hunan Medical College, 1958(1):48

16. Gupta D. Indian Medical Gazette 1929 64:67

17. Seery TM et al., J Pharmacology and Experimental Therapeutics 1940, 69:64

18. Zheng WF, Chinese Medical J 1952, 38:315

19. Sun X. Chinese Medical J 1955 41(6):536

20. Petlychna LI et al., BA 1977, 63(7):40192

21. Schmitz H. CA 1952, 463159e

22. Hirsch HH, CA 1953, 47:2888i

23. Meisel NM et al., CA 1958, 52:5535f

24. Luchnik NV, CA 1962,67:4985f

25. Borodina VM, Iidr: Tsitologiia 1977, 19(9):1067

26. Tang RY et al., Chinese Medical J 1958, 44(2):150

27. Zhu Y. Pharmacology and Applications of Chinese Medicinal Materials, People's Medical Publishing House, 1958, P.12

28. Turova AD et al., CA 1963, 58:2763b

29. Velluda CC et al., CA 1959, 53:15345a

30. Vartazaryan BA et al., CA 1965,62:15304g

31. Hahn FE et al., Antibiotics, Vol. III. JW Corcoran and FE Hahn, Springer-Verlag, Berlin, 1975. p.577

32. Sabit M et al., Indian J physiology and Pharmacology, 1971 15(3):111

33. Sadritdinov F. CA 1967 66:74714v

34. Jin DF, Acta Academica Medicinae Sichuan, Special Edition on Comprehensive Studies of Coptis, 1959 (1):102

35. 302nd Hospital of the Chinese PLA. Chinese J of Internal Medicine, 1976 new 1(4):219

36. Turova AD et al., CA 1964, 61:15242f

37. Hanzhou 2nd Medial College, Bulletin of Chinese Materia Medica 1958, 4(11):384

38. Ji YB, Pharmacological Action and Application of Available Composition of TCM, Helongjiang Science and Technology Press, 1994, pp.69-80

VII-8: Cordyceps Capsule

Constituent Herb and its Traditional Use

Cordyceps sinensis is known as *dong chong xia cao* in Chinese. It is the stroma of *Cordyceps sinensis* (Berk.) Sacc. (Ascomycetes) together with the host larva of *Hepialus armoricanus Oberthur* (*Hepialidae*).[1] Originally, it was found only in a small area of Qinghai province of China. Since it is very rare and expensive, Chinese scientists have found a way to cultivate it and make it more accessible. The cultivated version is made from the dried mycelia powder of *Cephalosporium sinensis Chen.*, isolated from fresh *Cordyceps sinensis* (Berk.) Sacc. through submerged fermentation in a liquid medium. [2]

TCM considers cordyceps warm-propertied with a sweet, acrid taste. It is lung-nourishing; kidney-, vital-essence- and vital-energy-tonifying; and phlegm-resolving. It is used to improve overall health following a prolonged illness, as well as to enhance the quality of life in the elderly.[1]

Chemical Composition

Cordyceps contains 17 amino acids, 10 trace elements, D-mannitol, and ergosterol. [3,4,5,6]

Pharmacology

The Beijing Institute of Material Medica of the Chinese Medical Academy made extensive pharmacological studies and found that the cultivated version of cordyceps has the same chemical components and the same physiological effects as the natural product.[7,8]

- ❖ Effects on cardiovascular system: It can increase blood flow to the heart, slow heartbeat, and lower blood pressure.

- ❖ Cordyceps lowers serum TC and TG, increases HDL, lowers LDL and VLDL, and combats arteriosclerosis.[9,10,11]

- ❖ Cordyceps increases platelet cAMP and platelet count, as well as white, red, and lymph cell count.

- ❖ Cordyceps enhances non-specific immunity and increases the weight of the spleen and the liver. It can increase Th cell count, activate NK and macrophage activity, and enhance Ts cell activities.

- ❖ Cordyceps can suppress Lewis lung cancer at a rate of 30-50%, as well as cervical cancer cells in culture.

- ❖ Cordyceps has sedative effects on the central nervous system.

- ❖ Cordyceps can dilate the air-ways of the lung and has shown anti-asthmatic effects.

❖ Its toxicity is very low and, in therapeutic
doses, there is virtually no toxicity. [12,13,14,15,16]

Clinical Applications

Cordyceps' superior therapeutic effects have been
confirmed in many controlled, well-designed studies
carried out by medical schools in Beijing, Shanghai,
Nanjing, and other major cities in China. Its therapeutic
effects to the liver have been extensively studied.

❖ In treating chronic viral hepatitis, the
effectiveness rate was above 80% in a 256-
patient clinical study. It can lower ALT,
improve liver function, relieve symptoms, and
increase albumin. It has also been used for
cirrhosis caused by viral hepatitis. In 22 cases,
after three months of use, 17 saw albumin
increase. Among 17 patients with ascites, 12
cases' ascites disappeared, while five cases
reduced their ascites. It can reduce enlarged
spleen and reduce pressure in the portal vein.
It can also dramatically improve stamina.

❖ Immune deficiency caused by viral infection,
chemotherapy, radiotherapy, or conditions
after major sicknesses and operations can be
improved with cordyceps.

❖ Chronic respiratory track infections, asthma,
bronchitis, and tuberculosis can be treated

with cordyceps and the flu and common cold can be prevented.

❖ Impotence, premature ejaculation, low libido, low sperm count and activity, irregular menstruation, and leucorrhoea can all be treated with cordyceps.

❖ Constitutional weakness due to cancer, AIDS, TB, convalescence, and wasting syndrome is improved with cordyceps.

❖ High blood lipoproteins and hypertension are alleviated with cordyceps.

❖ Cordyceps can be used to treat arrhythmia. It can accelerate atrioventricular conduction, enhance or regulate sinus rhythm, inhibit ectopic rhythm, and improve heart function.

Packaging and Dosage

Each capsule contains 300mg of Cordyceps sinensis mycelium, and each bottle contains 90 capsules. Take two tablets three times a day before meals.

References

1. The Great Dictionary of Chinese Materia Medica, Shanghai Science and Technology Press, 1988, p.767-768

2. Wang GD et al., Cordyceps, Its ecology, Cultivation, and Applications, Science and Technology Literature Press, 1995

3. Tang TH, Bulletin of Chinese Society of Pharmaceutics. 1947, 3(1):1

4. Sprecher M. et al., J. Org Chem 1963, 28:2490

5. Miyazake, et al., Chem Pharm Bull, 1977, (25):435

6. Liu RJ et al, Bulletin of Pharmaceutics, 1981, 16:567

7. Institute of Materia Medica of Chinese Medical Academy, Modern Studies of Chinese Materia Medica, Vol. 1, 1995, pp.91-112

8. Yang YP et al., Medicinal Fungi, 1986, 1:18

9. Bao TT et al., Chinese J Inte Traditional and Western Medicine, 1988, 8:352

10. Li L et al., Pharmacology and Clinics of Chinese Materia Medica, 1992, 8:6

11. Lou YQ et al., Chinese Herbs, 1986,17:209

12. Zhao YJ et al., Chinese J of Medicine, 1991, 71:612

13. Fun MG et al., Communication of Chinese Parmacology, 1989, 6:101

14. Zao G et al., Chinese J Inte Traditional and Western Medicine, 1985, 5:652

15. Yang WZ et al., Jiangxi TCM, 1985, (5):46

16. Zhrng FR, Chinese J of Hospital Pharmacy, 1992, 12:84

VII-9: R-5081 Capsule

Constituent Herbs

Smilax glabra, Scutellariae radix, Coptis chinensis Franch radix, Taraxaci Herba, Lonicerae Flos, Polygoni cuspidati rhizoma, and *Glycyrrhiza uralensis.*

Pharmacology

The phytopharmacology of the major ingredients of this formula—*Smilax glabra, Scutellariae radix, Coptis chinensis* Franch *radix,* and *Glycyrrhiza uralensis* are presented here.

❖ *Smilax glabra* root has been successfully used for treating syphilis and leptospirosis, and has been studied as a preventative treatment for leptospirosis. In 2,000 people tested, the incident rate of a pre-treated group compared with a control group was 1:5.58, a statistically significant result, demonstrating that taking the herb can successfully prevent leptospirosis. When used to treat syphilis, *S. glabra* combined with other Chinese herbs can achieve a greater than 90% cure rate. Even for the late stages of syphilis, the cure rate is above 50%. [1]

❖ *Scutellariae radix* has been effectively used to treat leptospirosis in China. [2]

❖ *Coptis chinensis* Franch radix major chemical ingredient is umbellatine. Pharmacological studies found it has a wide anti-infectious spectrum. It can strongly suppress *Staphylococcus aureus, Streptococc, pneumococcus, Vibrio comma, Anthrax bacillus,* and *Bacillus dysenteriae.* It can also suppress *Hay bacillus, Pneumobacillus, Bacillus diphtheriae, Bordetella pertussis, Brucellaceae,* and *Mycobacterium tuberculosis.* Its potency is roughly equal to or stronger than that of sulfanilamide and slightly weaker than that of streptomycin and chloramphenicol. It can suppress influenza viruses and Newcastle disease virus, as well as *Chlamydi trachomatis, trichomonad,* and *Leptospira.* Its toxicity is low; it has virtually no side effects. Long-term use has not caused any adverse reactions and no accumulative toxicity. LD_{50} for rats is 205mg/kg. [3,4,5,6,7,8,9]

❖ *Glycyrrhiza uralensis* (Licorice root) has anti-allergic, anti-inflammatory, and detoxifying activities-all important in treating chronic LD. Further, it promotes the regeneration of inflammatory tissue, in contrast with glucocorticoid, which inhibits regeneration. It also inhibits the release of histamine from mast cells, thus reducing inflammation. [10]

Packaging and Dosage

One capsule contains 750 mg of the extract of this formula. One bottle contains 45 capsules. Take one capsule three times a day before meals.

References

1. The Great Dictionary of Chinese Materia Medica, Shanghai Science and Technology Press, 1988, p.91-93

2. The Great Dictionary of Chinese Materia Medica, Shanghai Science and Technology Press, 1988, p.2017-2021

3. Xu ZL, Chinese Medical Journal, 1947, 33:71

4. Chen MR, Acta Academiae Medicinae Sichuan (Special Edition on Comprehensive Studies of Coptis) 1955 (1):55

5. Xu ZL, Acta Academiae Medicinae Sichuan (Special Edition on Comprehensive Studies of Coptis) 1955 (1):41

6. Gao SY et al., Science 1949, 110(1):11

7. Liao YX, Acta Pharmaceutica Sinica, 1954, 2(1):5

8. Zhao CY et al., Acta Microbiologica Sinica 1960, (8):171

9. Amin AH et al., Canadian J of Microbiology, 1969,15:1067

10. The Great Dictionary of Chinese Materia Medica, Shanghai Science and Technology Press, 1988, p.567-573

VII-10: HerbSom Capsule

HerbSom Capsule is made from the extracts of an herbal formula used for hundreds of years in China for improving sleep.

Constituent Herbs

Corydalis yanhusao rhizoma,[1] *Zizyphus spinosi semen,* [2] and *Schizandrae fructus.*[3]

Pharmacology

In a 374-patient study, improvement in sleep induced by HerbSom was found to be statistically equivalent to that of methaqualone, an insomnia drug, but without adverse reactions. It is not habit-forming and has no hangover effect. Pharmacological data on HerbSom's constituent herbs show that they benefit the cardiovascular and neurological systems. These herbs have no harmful effects on the liver and indeed are used to treat liver disease. [4]

Packaging and Dosage

Each capsule contains 300mg of the extracts of HerbSom Formula, with 60 capsules per bottle, enough for one month. Take two capsules at bedtime. **Do not take while driving a car or operating heavy machinery.**

References

1. The Great Dictionary of Chinese Materia Medica, Shanghai Science and Technology Press, 1988, p.919-922

2. The Great Dictionary of Chinese Materia Medica, Shanghai Science and Technology Press, 1988, p.2534-2536

3. The Great Dictionary of Chinese Materia Medica, Shanghai Science and Technology Press, 1988, p.386-389

4. Ma YD et al., Chinese J Of Integrated Traditional and Western Medicine, 1989, 9(2):85-87

VII-11: HH Capsule

Constituent Herb

Houttuyniae herba is the leaf of *Houttuynia cordata Thunb. (Saururaceae).* [1]

Pharmacology

The chief anti-bacterial compound of *H. cordata* is decanoyl acetaldehyde. [2,3,4]

HH has been effectively used to prevent and treat leptospirosis, an infectious disease caused by spirochetes. [5]

HH has shown significant activity against many bacteria and fungi. *In vitro* tests showed that it could markedly inhibit gram-positive and gram-negative bacteria. The most sensitive organisms were *Staphylococcus aureus* and its penicillin-resistant strains, *Diplococcus pneumoniae, Alpha streptococcus, Hemophilus influenzae. Neisseria catarrhalis,* and *Salmonella typhi. Escherichia coli, Pseudomonas aeruginosa,* and *Shigella dysenteriae* showed marginal sensitivity. [5,6,7, 8]

HH also inhibits *Candida albicans, Cryptococcus neoformans, Sporotruichum, Aspergillus, Chromomycosis, Epidermophyton rubrum, Tinea imbricata, Microsporum gypseum, Microsporum ferrugineum,* and *sharkskin fungus.* HH has shown

inhibitory action against *Diplococcus pneumoniae,
Salmonella typhi, Staphylococcus aureus, Escherichia
coli* and *Sporotrichum in vitro.* It has also strong
inhibitory action against *Mycobacterium tuberculosis*
both in vitro and in vivo. HH injection to tuberculin mice
at 1mg/mouse prolonged survival by 62 days; the
therapeutic effect was enhanced when the agent was
mixed with the animal feed. [9,10]

HH is also immune-enhancing, edema-alleviating, and
anti-inflammatory, all of which are of great importance
in the treatment of infectious diseases. [11,12]

Pharmacokinetic studies found that its half-life is 3.5
hours in rat gastrointestinal tract. It was quickly
distributed, first in the lungs, next in the heart, liver,
and kidneys, and minimally in the serum. [13]

HH has very low toxicity. The LD_{50} in mice was 1.6±
0.81 g/kg. Intravenous infusion of 38 or 47 mg/kg to
dogs did not cause any abnormalities in the heart, lungs,
liver, kidneys, spleen, stomach, or intestines.[14]

Clinical Applications

* Leptospirosis [15,16] and Lyme disease

* Respiratory tract infections [17,18]

* Chronic cervicitis [19]

* Otorhinolaryngological infections [20]

Packaging and Dosage

Each capsule contains 90mg of decanoyl acetaldehyde and absorbing substance. One bottle contains 45 tablets. Take one capsule three times a day.

References

1. The Great Dictionary of Chinese Materia Medica, Shanghai Science and Technology Press, 1988, p.1439-1441

2. Liu YL et al., Pharmaceutical Abstracts. Chinese Pharmaceutical Association (Beijing Branch). Sept 1978. p.231

3. Kosuge T. J of the Pharmaceutical Society of Japan (Tokyo) 1975, 72(10):1227

4. Isogai Y. C. A. 1953, 47:2832a

5. Leptospirosis Research Unit, Chengdu College of Traditional Chinese Medicine. Scientific Research Compilation. 3rd edition, Chengdu College of TCM, 1972. p.59

6. Yang HC et al., C A. 1953 47:8175d

7. Leptospirosis Research Unit, Sichuan Institute of Chinese Materia Medica. Research Information on TCM, 1971 (6):34

8. Jiangxi Medical Information (Jiangxi School of Pharmacy), 1972 (2):12

9. Kosuge T et al.,, . J of the Pharmaceutical Society of Japan (Tokyo) 1953, 73(5):435; 1956 76(4):386; 74(8):819;

10. Materia Medica Section, Bateriology-Immunology Dept. Beijing Institute of

Tuberculosis. Pharmaceutical Abstracts. Chinese Pharmaceutical Association, 1978, p.264

11. Bronchitis Unit, Third People's Hospital of Shanghai Second Medical College. J of TCM, 1973 (7):25

12. Medical Laboratory, Teaching Hospital of Jiangxi College of TCM, New Medical Information, 1975 (2):46

13. Materia Medica Unit, Jiangxi Second people's Hospital. Chinese J of Medicine, 1976 56(7):454

14. Jiangxi College of TCM, New Medical Information, 1977 (1):38

15. Liang YQ, Heilongjiang Medical J 1978(5):22

16. TCM Dept. Chengdu College of TCM, Acientific research Compilation. 4th edition, 1975, p.6

17. Pediatrics Dept, Fujian People's Hospital. Medical Information of Fuzhou Institute of Medical Science, 1975 (2):62

18. Zhong CY, People Military Medicine 1979 (3):39

19. Qui CQ et al., New Chinese Medicine 1979 10(12):601

20. Ji HK et al., J of TCM 1979 (5):28

VII-12: Puerarin Capsule

Constituent Herb

It is the root of *Pueraria thomsanii* Bent, or *P. lobata* Wild. Its Chinese name is *Ge Gen* whcih is considered by TCM to be mild-propertied with a sweet, pungent taste. It is fever-reducing, anti-spasm, and anti-diarrhea. It is also thought to induce the eruption of measles at the early stage. This herb is used in TCM to treat fever, headache, stiff back and neck, dry mouth in diarrhea or dysentery, and early-stage measles. [1]

Pharmacology

❖ Coronary and cerebral vasodilatory effects: Intravenous injection of puerarin in anesthetized dogs decreased heart rate, slightly decreased left ventricular work, reduced myocardial oxygen consumption, and increased myocardial efficiency. Cardiac output, however, was not significantly altered. These effects were beneficial to the maintenance of equilibrium between myocardial oxygen demand and supply [2, 3]. IV injection of extract of *Ge Gen* in anesthetized dogs with acute myocardial infarction caused significant decrease in blood pressure, slowing of heart beat, and slight decrease in blood flow in the infarcted area. At the same time, it caused no significant change in the arterial blood oxygen, but significant increase in the venous blood oxygen at the coronary sinus and infarcted area. Oxygen utilization and consumption, as well as lactic acid content, in both the normal and infarcted areas, were markedly decreased, whereas lactic acid utilization was markedly increased. These results indicate that puerarin has excellent effects on the metabolism of infarcted myocardium [4]. Injection of total puerarin flavones to the internal carotid artery of anesthetized dogs caused a dose-dependent increase in cerebral blood flow and a decrease in cerebral vascular resistance [5].

❖ Hypotensive effects: The herb can lower blood pressure, thereby explaining its effectiveness in treating migraines.[3, 5, 6]

❖ Inhibition of platelet aggregation: ADP-induced rat platelet aggregation was inhibited to different extents by 0.25, 0.5, and 1.0 mg/ml of puerarin *in vitro* and by intravenous injection. At doses of 0.5-3.0mg/ml, puerarin also inhibited aggregation of rabbit and sheep platelets, and those of normal subjects induced by ADP or serotonin. [7] These effects make it both a preventative measure and a treatment for angina pectoris and myocardial infarction.

❖ Studies have shown that, following administration, puerarin is rapidly distributed and eliminated, with low accumulation. [8] Oral administration of dried ethanol extract (10,000-20,000 mg/kg daily for three days) to mice did not result in any toxic effects. LD_{50} of the dried ethanol extract in mice was 2,100±120 mg/kg. Oral administration of the ethanol extract (2,000 mg/kg daily) to mice for two months did not cause pathological changes in the solid organs. Likewise, administration of the ethanol extract to hypertensive dogs (2,000 mg/kg daily for 14 days) produced no toxic effects.[9]

Clinical Applications

❖ Headache and migraine: Symptomatic improvement was achieved in 35 of 42 migraine cases. [9] In hypertensive patients, cerebral blood flow improved, vascular resistance decreased, and influx time was reduced in about 50% of the cases. [2, 9, 10]

❖ Coronary disease and angina pectoris: 191 cases of coronary disease and angina pectoris were treated with *Ge Gen* tablet, three or four tablets three times a day. This treatment was effective in relief of angina and in improving ECG [2,9,11]. Another group of 110 cases of coronary disease were treated with a compound of extract of puerarin and crataegi; 90% of them had relief of angina and 43% had marked improvement. [12]

❖ Sudden deafness: Tablets of the ethanol extract of *Ge Gen* (each equivalent to 1.5g of the crude herb) were used at a dose of one to two tablets three times a day together with injection of the total flavones, 100mg IM twice daily (and in some cases also supplemented with vitamin B complex), to treat 176 cases for a course of one to two months. Hearing improved in 79.5% of the cases. [2, 9, 13]

Packaging and Dosage

Each capsule contains 350mg of the extract of *Ge Gen* and about 100mg total flavones and puerarin. Each bottle contains 90 capsules, for a half month's supply. Take two tablets three times daily before meals.

References

1. Fang QC et al., Chinese Medical Journal 1974 (5):271

2. Institute of Materia Medica of Chinese Academy of Medical Sciences. Medical Research Communications 1972 (2):14

3. Fan LL et al., Chinese Medical Journal 1975 (10):724

4. Zhou YP et al., Chinese Medical Journal 1977 (9):550

5. Zeng GY et al., Chinese Medical Journal 1974 (5):265

6. Zeng GY et al., Chinese Medical Journal 1979 (8):479

7. Pharmacology Department, Institute of Materia Medica of the Chinese Academy of Medical Sciences, Research Information on Cardiovascular Diseases 1979 (12):1

8. Zhu XY et al., Acta Pharmaceutica Sinica 1979 14(6):349

9. Institute of Materia Medica of the Chinese Academy of Medical Sciences, Chinese Traditional and Herbal Drugs Communications 1975 (2):34

10. Hypertension Research Unit, Fuwai Hospital of the Chinese Academy of Medical Sciences, Cardiovascular Diseases 1972 (1):29

11. Beijing Railways Hospital et al., Proceedings of the Symposium of Stage-IV Research Summary of Beijing Distract Coordinating Research Group on Coronary Diseases 1972 (2):36

12. Anshan P Pharmaceutical Factory, Chinese Traditional and Herbal Drugs Communications 1978 (2):20

13. Auditus Department, Beijing Institute of Otorhinoloryngology, Chinese Medical Journal 1973 (10):591

Appendix 1
The Safety of Artemisia

One of the most important discoveries in the modernization movement of TCM was the anti-malarial effect of artemisia's active ingredient, arteannuin or artemisinin, which has been exhaustively studied for more than 30 years in China. What follows is a review of artemisia's anti-malarial effects and clinical applications. In order to improve the anti-malarial efficacy and reduce relapse rate and toxicity, many more effective, safer derivatives of arteannuin have been developed, and the original form of the active ingredient is no longer in clinical use.

Pharmacokinetics

Following oral administration of ^{3}H-arteannuin in mice, blood radioactivity peaked in 0.5-1 hour, and in equally rapid fashion, descended to below the half-peak value in 4 hours. Thereafter, the radioactivity disappeared slowly, and within 72 hours, only small amounts were left in the body. Its distribution was most abundant in the kidneys and liver, followed, in descending order by the heart, lungs, spleen, muscles, bones, and brain. Within 24 hours, 56.3±9.8% of the radioactivity was excreted in the urine and 22.2±2.3% in the feces; the total excretion was 80%. Thirty minutes after intravenous injection, arteannuin in the blood was mostly metabolized; most of the substance excreted in the urine consisted of metabolites. [1,2] On the cellular level, the concentration of arteannuin in *Plasmodium*-infected red cells was 100 times higher than non-infected cells. Obviously, this distribution pattern made it easier to contact the *Plasmodium* parasites and made it more effective as an anti-malarial agent. [3] Because it can rapidly penetrate the BBB, it is currently the most effective treatment for brain malaria. The rate of arteannuin oral absorption $T_{1/2}$ was one hour. [4, 5]

Metabolites of orally administered arteannuin in human urine consisted of hydroarteannuin and reduced hydroarteannuin. They were devoid of anti-malarial activity in rats, suggesting that the metabolism of arteannuin is an inactivation process. [6] In conclusion, the pharmacokinetic characteristics of arteannuin are rapid absorption, wide distribution, rapid penetration of the BBB, rapid metabolism and excretion, and absence of accumulation.

Acute Toxicity and Therapeutic Index

LD_{50}, ED_{50}, and therapeutic index (LD_{50}/ED_{50}) within three days of observation of the various preparations of the herb are listed in the following table. [1]

Acute Toxicity and Anti-malarial Therapeutic Index of *Qing hao* Preparations

Preparation	LD_{50}(mg/kg)	ED_{50}(mg/kg)	Therapeutic Index (LD_{50}/ED_{50})
Neutral fraction of ether extract	7425	2646	2.80
Dilute alcohol extract	4162	2526	1.64
Arteannuin (Artemisinin)	5105	139	36.80
Reduced arteannuin	465	33	14.10

*In comparison, the therapeutic index of chloroquine is 28.8.

The LD_{50} of the oil suspension of arteannuin by intramuscular and intraperitoneal injections and of the aqueous suspension by subcutaneous injection were 2800, 1558, and over 9000 mg/kg, respectively. [2]

The LD_{50} of arteannuin for mice by intra-stomach administration was 4223mg/kg, therapeutic index was 47.1, and safety index was 13.7. Animal tests using cats, rabbits, dogs, rats, mice, and guinea pigs, and administration through stomach, intramuscular injection, and intraperitoneal injection, with dosages of 100-1600mg/kg—70 times clinical dose—continuously administrated for 3 to 7 days, found no changes in the general health status, appetite, weight, and cardiovascular, liver, and kidney functions.[2]

When the active anti-malarial constituent, arteannuin, was given to healthy dogs at an increased dosage of 2,000 mg/kg, four out of 10 dogs showed higher SGPT activity than normal. After intragastric administration of arteannuin to mice at the dose of 800 mg/kg for 3 days, a transient elevation of GPT was observed on the 4th and 8th days. Cloudy swelling of liver cells and petechia in the brain were seen in pathologic sections, but no significant changes in the morphology and function of other organs. [1, 2, 7, 8] When arteannuin was given orally to patients at the dose of 3,000mg twice daily for 3 days, or in gradually increasing doses up to 5,000 mg daily, individual patients developed abdominal pain and occult blood in stool. One patient given the dose of 5,000 mg had elevated transaminase level. Oral administration of 3,000-5,000 mg to a man for 3 days did not produce significant alterations in the EKG, EEG, liver, or renal function tests, or chest X-ray, or in routine urine and blood examinations. One out of 3 cases developed numbness of the extremities and another had tachycardia, but all recovered quickly.[1] In conclusion, *qing hao* and arteannuin are low in acute toxicity.

Sub-acute and Long-term Toxicity

Tests on dogs and rats by intramuscular injections at a dose of 40mg/kg/day for 14 days and tests on mice by oral administration at a dose of 2400-3400 mg/kg/day and intramuscular injection at a dose of 800mg/kg/day for 3 days found no histological changes in major organs. [9]

The ultrastructure of the cardiac muscle of monkey, intramuscularly injected with arteannuin at a dose of 96mg/kg/day for 16 days, started showing submicroscopic damage, which was reversible after the drug was stopped. [10]

In a sub-acute toxicity study, dogs and rats taking 70 times the clinical dose for 21 days experienced no changes in EEG, EKG, liver function, blood count, total protein, appetite, or growth. Only in dogs were elevation in non-protein nitrogen and reversible histological changes in heart, liver, and kidneys exhibited. [2]

Efficacy and Toxicity of Derivatives of Arteannuin

In recent years, many studies have been done to improve solubility and efficacy in treating malaria, to reduce relapse rate, and to further lower toxicity. To these ends, arteannuin's molecular structure has been altered and derivatives have been developed.

Arteannuin is a sesquiterpene lactone, which has a peroxide group. Hydrogenation or treatment with acid or alkaline of the peroxide group resulted in the loss of anti-malarial activity of arteannuin. A reduced arteannuin, obtained by reduction of the carboxyl group on the 12th carbon into a hydroxyl group, exhibited a significantly higher anti-malarial effect and toxicity. [1] To overcome the problems of high relapse rate, low solubility, and difficulty in preparing the injection liquid of arteannuin, the reduced arteannuin was used as a base and the H of the hydroxyl group on the 12th carbon was replaced with a different group to form a lactone compound from which several derivatives were obtained with even stronger anti-malarial activity. In terms of anti-malarial activity, toxicity, stability, and cost, the following three derivatives were considered ideal: SM 224($-CH_3$(b)), SM 242($-CO-CH_2CH_2CH_3$ (a)), and SM 108($-CO-CH_2-CH_3$(a)). The efficacy of these agents was more than tenfold that of arteannuin. They were effective against chloroquine-resistant strains, less toxic, and more fat-soluble. In monkey malaria, no relapse was noted during the 81-day follow-up period after a sufficient dose of SM 224 or SM 108. [11]

Another derivative--804-Na($-CO-CH_2 CH_2-COO-Na$)--was very water-soluble and had a better anti-malarial activity in rats than arteannuin. Intraperitoneal injection of this agent at 120 mg/kg, or oral administration at 240 mg/kg, for 3 days cured all the infected animals, and no relapse was detected within 35 days. The maximal tolerable dose in mice was 225 times the human dose. There were no adverse reactions to the intravenous or intramuscular injection of the aqueous preparation. [12, 13]

Specific Toxicity for Arteannuin and its Derivatives

Arteannuin as an anti-malarial has a very low toxicity, though a frequent adverse reaction is transient suppression of reticulocytes, which spontaneously return to normal once treatment is suspended.[14] In animal studies, it has shown fetal toxicity during the fetal organ development stage, though it didn't cause any birth defects. These effects have not been studied in humans, though a retrospective analysis in a clinical setting found that babies born to women who were taking arteannuin during pregnancy had no birth defects. [15, 16] To be on the safe side, however, arteannuin and its derivatives should not be used during the first trimester of pregnancy.

Mice teratogenetic studies found that arteannuin did not affect normal fetal development and birth.[17] Arteannuin was proved in experiments to have no teratogenic effect and no effect on the sperm of mice. [18] Mutogenicity tests found that it was not a mutagen and has no oncogenitic effects. [19]

Neurological toxicity was found using derivatives of arteannuin at a high dose of 20mg/kg/day, which is 15-18 times higher than the clinical dose of 80mg/day, for 5 days in rats and 9 days in dogs. Histological changes occurred in the brain, with damage mostly in the pons and medulla oblongata. The most pronounced changes were neuron degeneration. When given doses of less than 20mg/kg/day, no neurological toxicity or histological changes were observed. [20, 21] Arteannuin has been replaced by newer, more effective, less toxic derivatives, such as artesunate, which has no reported neurological toxic side effects.[22]

Clinical Adverse Reactions

An important characteristic of artemisia is its low toxicity. Of 590 malarial patients treated with a tablet of the herbal extract, only 3.4% developed gastrointestinal symptoms such as nausea, vomiting, abdominal pain, and diarrhea. [23] Another 2,089 cases treated with various preparations of arteannuin showed no significant side effects: 139 of these cases had CPT and ECG examined before and after treatment, and 75 examined for non-protein nitrogen; no abnormalities were discovered. The herb did not produce any adverse effects in patients with heart, liver, or kidney disease, or in pregnant women. Only mild pain over the injection site after the intramuscular dose of the aqueous suspension was reported. [2] A few cases of allergic reactions were reported when arteannuin was used as an injective. [24] The use of newer derivatives of arteannuin, such as artesunate, has greatly improved therapeutic efficacy and safety, and further reduced adverse reactions.

Conclusion

Artemisia has been used in TCM for thousands of years. It has long been known to have anti-malarial effects. During the modernization of TCM, its anti-malarial ingredient, arteannuin, was isolated and purified. For more than 30 years, this substance's pharmacology, pharmacokinetics, toxicity, and clinical applications have been extensively studied. It has been found to have very low toxicity and can be used safely as an anti-malarial agent. In order to reduce relapse rate and further reduce its toxicity, many derivatives have been developed. At the therapeutic dosage, only 3.4% of cases develop gastrointestinal symptoms such as nausea, vomiting, abdominal pain, and diarrhea, and transient reduction of reticular erythrocyte. All these adverse reactions are reversible upon cessation of treatment stopped. In conclusion, this is a very safe and effective remedy.

References

1. Pharmacology Department, Institute of Chinese Materia Medica of the Academy of Traditional Chinese Medicine. Xinyiyaoxue Zazhi (Journal of Traditional Chinese Medicine) 1979 (1):23.

2. Coordinating Research Group on Qinghao. Chinese Pharmaceutical Bulletin 1979; 14 (2): 49.

3. Gu HM et al., Transactions of The Royal Society of Tropical Medicine and Hygiene, 1984; 78:265

4. Chen R et al., J New TCM, 1979; (6) :51

5. Chen R et al., J New TCM, 1980; (1):37

6. Institute of Materia Medica, Chinese Academy of Sciences. Metabolites of Arteannuin (internal information).1978.

7. Li S. et al., New Traditional Chinese Medicine, 1979; (6):51

8. Li S. et al., New Traditional Chinese Medicine, 1980; (1):37

9. Zhou JH et al., Pharmacology of Chinese Materia Medica, Shanghai Science and Technology Press, 1986

10. Wu WD et al., Chinese Pharmaceutical Bulletin 1983; 4(3):191

11. Institute of Materia Medica, Chinese Academy of Sciences. Synthesis and pharmacological studies of arteannuin derivatives (abstract) (internal information). 1978.

12. Guangxi Medical College et al. Preliminary studies on the pharmacology of 804-Na, a derivative of arteannuin (internal information). 1978.

13. Liu X. Chinese Pharmaceutical Bulletin 1980 15(4):39.

14. Wu BA et al., J. Chinese Clinical Pharmacology, 1987; 3:156

15. Li ZL et al., J. Chinese Clinical Pharmacology, 1985; 1 (supple):28

16. Chen LJ et al., Chinese Pharmaceutical J. 1980 15(4):39.

17. Ke MQ The Physicochemical and Pharmacological Nature of the Active Ingredients of Chinese Herbs. Second edition, Hunan Science and Technology Press, 1982; 447

18. Liu T et al. Xinzhongyi (Journal of New Chinese Medicine) 1979 (6):5].; 1980 (1):37.

19. Li GY et al., J. of Traditional Chinese Medicine, 1981; 22 (6):67

20. Swearengen J et al., Transactions of The Rohal Society of Tropical Medicine and Hygiene, 1994; 88(suppl):33

21. Ning TX et al., Chinese J. Pharmacology and Toxicology, 1987;1:135

22. Lin BX et al., J. Hospital Pharmacy, 1982; (5):35

23. Sichuan Institute of Chinese Materia Medica (editor). Research Information on Chinese Traditional Drugs 1978 (l4):24,. 36..

24. Li ZQ et al., J New Medicine, 1985; 16(11):576

Appendix 2

Frequently Asked Questions about MCM Treatment of LD

How did you begin treating LD? How many cases have you treated?

We saw our first LD patients about 12 years ago and started by treating their muscular-skeletal pain with acupuncture. Many patients' pain could not be cured without treating their underlying LD, so we began researching how to treat LD with Chinese medicine. At first we borrowed the TCM treatments for syphilis, leptospirosis, and other spirochete diseases. Later we researched the phytopharmacology of Chinese herbs to match the pathology of LD. From this research, we gradually developed our treatment protocols.

Up to now, we have treated more than a thousand LD patients, mostly chronic or persistent LD sufferers. They were either non-responders to antibiotics, or could not tolerate antibiotics because of the side effects. We have also treated some acute LD infections with a much shorter treatment course.

Do you have a vested interest in the herbs used at your clinic?

We use Chinese herbal remedies, which are not regulated by the FDA, so we personally ensure the potency and quality of the herbal products used in our clinic. We design the formulas, supervise their manufacture, and distribute them. We use our name as the brand name.

How long will it take to get an appointment with you? How long will the first consultation last?

It usually takes two to three weeks to get an appointment. The first consultation will last about one hour.

What is your philosophy of an appropriate treatment strategy?

A proper treatment strategy should address the entire pathophysiological problem of a disease. In LD, merely combating the infectious pathogens with antibiotics is not sufficient because inadequate immune reactions must also be regulated. Indeed, most LD symptoms are the result of inadequate immune reactions, such as autoimmunity, which causes CNS and muscular-skeletal symptoms. Pathogen eradication is best accomplished by strengthening the body's immune response. Antibiotics do not do this.

Is your treatment covered by insurance?

The herbal remedies are not covered by insurance. Acupuncture treatments may be covered, depending on your policy.

Can MCM treatment eradicate the Lyme spirochete and co-infection pathogens?

Yes, MCM herbal treatments are curative treatments for Lyme disease and its co-infections. They do not merely suppress symptoms. They eradicate the pathogens and promote repair of damaged tissue. The majority of our patients have been staying symptom-free and their pathogen PCR test turned to negative following a complete course of the treatment.

How long is the MCM treatment course for chronic LD?

Treatment for acute LD is about two months, if the infection is diagnosed immediately following the tick bite. For chronic LD, however, the course is at least six months. For a very small number of patients, if their disease is very disseminated and the disease course has been very long, they may need ongoing treatment to control their symptoms.

What is your success rate in treating chronic LD?

We do not have a statistical analysis to answer this question exactly. From our clinical observations, however, we have seen at least 60% of our patients turn asymptomatic (without symptoms) following herbal treatment and more than 80% improved. Less than 20% of our patients have not responded to our herbal treatments. Because laboratory tests are not conclusive, we cannot definitely declare a patient is cured; therefore, these figures are only approximations.

Can MCM treat acute LD?

Yes, we have treated many patients who had just been bitten by ticks and didn't want to use antibiotics. For these patients, the treatments were mainly anti-*Babesia* and anti-spirochete herbs, which have a wide spectrum of anti-microbial effects and so can also address co-infections other than babesiosis. The treatment course was about two months. If they caught the infection early and started treatment right away, their LD did not become chronic.

Can MCM treatment be used concurrently with Western medical treatment?

Yes, MCM herbal protocols can be used alone or together with Western antibiotics. No adverse interaction has been observed.

Can MCM treatment be a stand-alone treatment for LD?

For patients who cannot tolerate antibiotics, MCM herbal treatment can be used as a stand-alone treatment. For those patients suffering from antibiotic-induced liver damage, evidenced in elevated liver enzymes ALT and AST, we have very effective herbal treatments to heal the liver. For patients already using antibiotics who want to taper off, we suggest using herbs concurrently with antibiotics at first and then, when the herbal effects kick in, gradually tapering off the antibiotics.

Can children use MCM for LD?

Yes, we have treated pediatric LD patients with MCM. The youngest was a year old. Because these herbal remedies have low toxicity, they are safe for children. The dose has to be adjusted for age and body weight. For children younger than 6 years, the dose is one-third the adult dose; for patients aged 6 to 12, the dose is half the adult dosage. Above 12 years old, the dose is the same as for an adult. If children cannot swallow the capsule, it can be opened and the contents mixed with food.

How do you determine an endpoint for MCM treatment?

This is a difficult question to answer. Blood tests are not accurate enough to determine whether the infection is still present. We must rely more heavily on presentation of symptoms than on blood tests. If after six months of treatment, the patient's symptoms are almost gone, then we encourage him or her to take a PCR (polymerase chain reaction) test. If it is negative, then we stop the treatment to observe the patient for one to two months. If the symptoms do not come back, we consider the treatment is completed.

Are there any side effects or adverse reactions?

Because of their low toxicity, MCM herbal remedies do not cause serious side effects. Herxheimer's reaction is a necessary part of healing, which is not considered an adverse reaction and is not caused by herbal toxicity. The only problem with one of the most important herbal remedies, allicin, is its strong garlic odor. Also for people with very sensitive stomachs, herbs may cause discomfort. Taking the herbs with food can reduce stomach irritation.

How do you control the quality of the herbal products?

First, we are using purified active ingredients, not the raw herbs; therefore, we can eliminate contaminants such as pesticides, fertilizers, and heavy metals. Moreover, when our products are exported from China and imported to the United States, they have to pass tests for heavy metals, pesticides, and bacterial content.

Second, the potency of our purified ingredients can be measured and calibrated. Our manufacturing practices meet the requirements of GMP (good manufacture practice) standard.

How expensive is MCM treatment?

Compared with conventional WM treatment, the herbs are very affordable—about one-twentieth of the cost of conventional medical treatment. But because herbs are not covered by insurance, and because many chronic LD patients are unable to work, the $2,000 or so for a complete treatment course may be difficult for some patients.

How do you monitor treatment progress?

We ask our patients to record their symptoms in a daily journal. Monitoring symptoms is our primary means of tracking disease regression and treatment progress. Once symptoms are no longer present, we encourage patients to take a PCR test to confirm the eradication of the pathogens.

If I cannot come to New York and want to take your herbal protocols, what should I do?

We provide phone consultation for people not living in New York. By reviewing your medical records and collecting your symptoms and signs over the phone, we determine what herbal formulas are right for you and have them sent by mail to your home. In this way, we even take care of patients in other countries.

How often do I need to visit your office during the MCM treatment course?

We usually see patients living in or near New York City at least two to three times in person, and then communicate through phone or email. The second visit is two weeks after the herbal treatment starts, because this time is the peak of Herxheimer's reaction, and patients usually have many questions. The third visit is about one month after this. If patients want acupuncture to supplement herbal treatment, then we see them once or twice a week.

Should I have regular acupuncture treatments?

Acupuncture is beneficial for improving brain function and relieving pain in the muscular-skeletal system. It also has immune-regulatory effects. Although it is not the major treatment for LD, it can be an important adjunctive treatment. If you can afford it or if your insurance pays for it, acupuncture should be done regularly.

How will acupuncture help treat my LD?

First, acupuncture can relieve joint and muscle aches and pain, which are major LD symptoms. Second, it can stimulate the brain to produce more beta-endorphin, which is a nature pain killer and it also helps regulate immune function. Third, it can improve brain function—something that has been confirmed through medical imaging techniques.

What is the difference between antibody tests, such as Western blot, and the polymerase chain reaction (PCR) test?

Antibodies are the proteins produced by the immune system to fight infectious microbials—the antigens. If an antibody test is positive, that means you have contracted the infection and your body has reacted to the infection by producing the specific antibodies that fight the invading microbial. These antibodies may be present even after the infection is cleared. Therefore, an antibody test cannot determine whether the infection is still present.

In contrast, PCR is an antigen test, which means it detects the presence of the DNA of the infectious pathogens. If it is positive, the pathogen is still present in your body, and you have an ongoing infection. At present, because both the antibody and antigen tests are not specific or sensitive enough, the results are not definite and do not allow us to make a conclusive diagnosis or a prognosis.

What diet do you recommend for people with chronic Lyme disease?

We recommend Dr. Andrew Weil's "anti-inflammatory diet" for people with chronic Lyme disease. He believes that diet influences inflammation and the food choices a person makes can determine whether who is in a proinflammatory state or in an anti-inflammatory one. Chronic LD is an inflammatory disorder and the anti-inflammatory diet is very suitable for patients with chronic LD. The principles to guide food choices are: "Aim for variety, and include as much fresh food as possible in your diet. Minimize your consumption of processed and fast food. Eat an abundance of fruits and vegetables, and try to include carbohydrates, fat and protein in every meal. Most adults need consume between 2,000 to 3,000 calories a day. ...The distribution of calories you take in should be: 40 to 50% from carbohydrates, 30% from fat and 20 to 30% from protein." For detailed information please visit www.healthyaging.com (Time, October 17, 2005, P.64, Dr. Andrew Weil's Wellness Diet)

Glossary

Acupuncture

A TCM treatment procedure in which specific points on the body associated with meridians and peripheral nerves are pierced with fine needles to produce analgesic effects and to promote blood and *qi* circulation. Acupuncture has been recommended by the World Health Organization to treat many chronic health conditions.

Allopathic

A method of treating disease with remedies that produce effects different from those caused by the disease itself. It often uses methods to suppress the disease manifestations. Western biomedicine is usually referred to as allopathic medicine.

Amebic dysentery

An acute disease caused by ingesting foods contaminated with the amoeba *Entamoeba histolytica* and characterized by severe diarrhea, nausea, and inflammation of the intestines.

Antibiotic

A substance, such as penicillin or streptomycin, produced by or derived from certain fungi, bacteria, and other organisms, that can destroy or inhibit the growth of other microorganisms. Antibiotics are widely used in the prevention and treatment of infectious diseases, mainly bacterial infections.

Antibiotic-resistant bacteria

Bacteria that cannot be suppressed or inhibited by antibiotics, though they were able to inhibit them before.

Antibodies

Y-shaped proteins on the surface of B cells that are secreted into the blood or lymph in response to an antigenic stimulus, such as a bacterium, virus, parasite, or transplanted organ, and that neutralize the antigen by binding specifically to it.

Anti-mitotic action

Preventing or interfering with mitosis (cell division).

Anti-neoplastic effects

Inhibiting or preventing the growth or development of tumors or malignant cells.

Anti-oxidant

A substance, such as vitamin E, vitamin C, or beta-carotene, thought to protect body cells from the damaging effects of oxidation caused by free radicals.

Appendicitis

Inflammation of the appendix.

Arteriosclerosis

A chronic disease in which thickening, hardening, and loss of elasticity of the arterial walls result in impaired blood circulation. It develops with aging, and in hypertension, diabetes, hyperlipidemia, and other conditions.

Auscultation

The act of listening for sounds made by internal organs to aid in diagnosis. In TCM the sounds of speech, coughing are also listened as one of the four diagnosis methods.

Autoimmunity

Of or relating to an immune response by the body against one of its own tissues, cells, or molecules.

Babesia

A genus of parasitic sporozoans of the family *Babesiidae* that infect the red blood cells of humans and of animals such as dogs, cattle, and sheep. Also called piroplasm.

Babesiosis or piroplasmosis

A human protozoan disease of red blood cells caused by Babesia species that is transmitted by the northern deer tick; characterized by fever, malaise, and hemolytic anemia; and prevalent in the northeastern United States. A common co-infection of Lyme disease that has spread to the Midwest and Pacific Coast.

Bacteria

Any of the unicellular prokaryotic microorganisms of the class Schizomycetes, which vary in terms of morphology, oxygen and nutritional requirements, and motility, and may be free-living, saprophytic, or pathogenic in plants or animals.

Bartonella

A genus of bacteria, *Bartonella bacilliformis*, found in humans and arthropods that multiply in red blood cells and endothelial cells and reproduce by binary fission. Cats commonly carry it, and its infection is usually caused by cat scratch; therefore, it is often called cat scratch disease. A common co-infection of LD.

Borrelia burgdorferi

A spirochete bacterium commonly carried by ticks, which can cause Lyme disease or borreliosis in humans and other warm-blooded animals.

Blood-brain barrier

A physiological protective mechanism that alters the permeability of brain capillaries, so that some substances are prevented from entering brain tissue, while other substances are allowed to enter freely.

Blood rheology

A study that investigates the liquidity of the blood, its viscosity, the clustering of blood cells, and the speed at which blood travels through the vessels.

Borreliosis

Disease caused by bacteria of the genus *Borrelia burgdorferi*.

Bell's palsy

An unilateral facial muscle paralysis of sudden onset, resulting from trauma, compression, or infection of the facial nerve and characterized by muscle weakness and a distorted facial expression.

Candidiasis

Infection with a fungus of the genus *Candida*, especially *C. albicans*, that usually occurs in the skin and mucous membranes of the mouth, respiratory tract, or vagina but may invade the bloodstream, especially in immune-compromised individuals.

Cellular immunity

Immunity resulting from a cell-mediated immune response that is carried by T-lymph cells.

Chemical precursor

A chemical substance, such as an intermediate compound in a chain of chemical reactions, from which another chemical is formed as the result of the reaction.

Chlorophyll

Any of a group of green pigments that are found in the chloroplasts of plants and in other photosynthetic organisms.

Chronic hepatitis

Inflammation of the liver lasting longer than six months or marked by frequent recurrence.

Circulatory immune complex (CIC)

Complexes of an antigen and an antibody in the blood.

Cirrhosis

A chronic liver disease characterized by the replacement of normal tissue with fibrous tissue and the loss of functional liver cells. It can result from alcohol abuse, nutritional deprivation, or infection especially by the hepatitis virus.

Co-infection

Concurrent infection of a cell, tissue, or organism with two or more microorganisms.

Cryptosporidiosis

A pathological condition caused by protozoa of the genus *Cryptosporidium* that infect humans and some animals, causing severe gastritis and diarrhea.

Cystic (dormant) form

In unfavorable conditions, a bacterium turned into a latent form, which is surrounded by a non-living membrane. It is capable of being activated when conditions improve.

Cytokines

Any of several regulatory proteins, such as the interleukins and lymphokines, that are released by cells of the immune system and act as intercellular mediators in the generation of an immune response.

Cytoskeleton

The internal framework of a cell.

Demyelination

Destruction or removal of the myelin sheath of a nerve fiber, as through some disease.

Diffuse intravenous coagulation or disseminated intravascular coagulation (DIC)

A pathological form of blood coagulation in the vein that is diffuse all over the body rather than localized.

ED_{50}

The effective dose on 50% of test subjects, used to indicate the efficacy of a medicinal substance.

Ehrlichia

A genus of bacteria of the *Rickettsiaceae* family that occurs singly or in circulating white blood cells and macrophage-monocytes.

Encephalopathy

A change of consciousness due to various diseases of the brain.

Endoerythrocytic protozoa

Protozoa occurring within red blood cells.

Endoplasmic reticulum

A membrane network within the cytoplasm of cells involved in the synthesis, modification, and transport of cellular materials.

Endorphin theory of acupuncture

Endorphins are released from brain into the bloodstream by the stimulation of acupuncture points to treat pain and complications of illness.

Erythema migrans

A spreading, red skin lesion that develops at the site of a tick bite and is an early sign of Lyme disease.

Fibroblasts

Cells that making collagen fibers and develop into connective tissue.

Fibromyalgia

A syndrome characterized by fatigue, tenderness at specific sites in the body, and chronic pain in the muscles and soft tissues surrounding the joints.

Functional magnetic resonance imaging (fMRI)

A form of magnetic resonance imaging that registers blood flow to functioning areas of the brain.

Fungi

Any of the numerous organisms of the kingdom Fungi, which lack chlorophyll and vascular tissue and range in form from a single cell to a body mass of branched *filamentous hyphae* that often produce specialized fruiting bodies. The kingdom includes yeasts, molds, smuts, and mushrooms.

Gate Theory

An acupuncture theory that suggests there are specific nerve fibers that transmit pain to the spinal cord, while other nerve fibers inhibit pain transmission, and that acupuncture excites the pain-inhibitory nerve fibers, thereby temporarily blocking the pain.

Granuloma

A mass of inflamed granulation tissue, usually associated with ulcerated infections.

Hematopoiesis

The formation of blood or blood cells in the body.

Hepatitis C

A liver infection caused by the hepatitis C virus and transmitted primarily by blood and blood contact, as in blood transfusions or intravenous drug use, though sometimes through sexual contact.

Herbology

The study of medicinal herbs.

Herxheimer's reaction

An inflammatory reaction in spirochete infections, such as LD and syphilis, induced by anti-spirochetal treatment with herbal remedies, salvarsan, mercury, or antibiotics.

Homeopathic

A system for treating disease based on the administration of minute doses of a drug that in massive amounts produces symptoms in healthy individuals similar to those of the disease itself.

Holistic

A system that focuses on the whole rather than on the component parts; TCM and MCM are holistic forms of medicine, whereas WM is not.

Human granulocytic ehrlichiosis (HGE)

A condition marked by fever, myalgia, headache, leucopoenia, and thrombocytopenia that is caused by a bacterium of the genus *Ehrlichia*, which is transmitted by ticks and infecting granulocytes (a type of white blood cell).

Human monocytic ehrlichiosis (HME)

A condition marked by fever, myalgia, headache, leucopoenia, and thrombocytopenia that is caused by a bacterium of the genus *Ehrlichia*, which is transmitted by ticks and infecting monocytes (a type of white blood cell).

Humeral immunity

An aspect of the immune system involving antibodies that are secreted by B lymph cells that circulate as soluble proteins in blood plasma and lymph.

IgG

The most abundant class of antibodies found in blood serum and lymph and which are active against bacteria, fungi, viruses, and foreign particles.

IgM

The class of antibodies found in circulating body fluids and the first to appear in response to an initial exposure to an antigen.

Immunity

Inherited, acquired, or induced resistance to infection by a specific pathogen or by foreign antigens.

Iatrogenic (medication-caused) disorders

Illness induced in a patient by a physician's activity, manner, or therapy.

Insomnia

Chronic inability to fall asleep or remain asleep for an adequate length of time.

Inquiring

TCM diagnostic method involving direct inquiry of the patient as to history of the disorder, nature of the symptoms, and response to treatment.

Inspection

TCM diagnostic method based on visual observation of the patient.

Irritable bowel syndrome

A disorder characterized by abnormally increased motility of the small and large intestines, producing abdominal pain, constipation, or diarrhea.

LD$_{50}$

The dose of a toxic agent or drug that is sufficient to kill 50% of a test population of animals within a certain time frame. It is used as an indicator of the toxicity of a substance.

Leprosy

A chronic, mildly contagious disease of tropical and subtropical regions, caused by the bacillus *Mycobacterium leprae*, characterized by ulcers of the skin, bone, and viscera, and leading to loss of sensation, paralysis, gangrene, and deformation. Also called Hansen's disease.

Leptospirosis

An infectious disease of human and domestic animals, especially cattle, swine, and dogs, caused by spirochetes of the genus *Leptospira*, characterized by jaundice, bleeding, and fever, and usually transmitted through contact with contaminated water.

Lymphocytes

Any of the nearly colorless cells found in the blood, lymph, and lymphoid tissues, constituting approximately 25% of white blood cells and including B cells, which function in humeral immunity, and T cells, which function in cellular immunity.

Macrophage

A large cell of the immune system whose function is to engulf and ingest bacteria or other foreign bodies.

Malaria

An infectious disease characterized by cycles of chills, fever, and sweating, caused by a protozoan of the genus *Plasmodium* in red blood cells, which is transmitted to humans by the bite of an infected female mosquito.

Megalokaryocyte

Giant bone-marrow cell that gives rise to upwards of 4,000 platelets.

Microcirculation

The flow of blood or lymph through the smallest vessels of the body.

Mitochondrial membrane

Thin, pliable layer of tissue covering the surface of the mitochondria of a cell.

Motion sickness

Nausea and dizziness induced by motion, as in travel by aircraft, car, or ship.

Multiple sclerosis (MS)

A chronic autoimmune disease of the central nervous system in which gradual destruction occurs throughout the brain or spinal cord or both, interfering with nerve pathways and causing muscular weakness, loss of coordination, and speech and visual disturbances.

Mycobacteria

Any of various slender, rod-shaped, aerobic bacteria of the genus *Mycobacterium*, which includes the bacteria that cause tuberculosis and leprosy.

Mycoplasma

Any of numerous parasitic, pathogenic microorganisms of the genus *Mycoplasma* that lack a true cell wall, are gram-negative, and need sterols such as cholesterol for growth. In humans, one species is a primary cause of nonbacterial pneumonia.

Myelin

A white, fatty material composed chiefly of lipids and lipoproteins that encloses certain axons and nerve fibers.

Neurotoxin

A toxin that damages or destroys nerve tissue.

Palpation

To examine or explore by touching an organ or area of the body for means of TCM diagnosis.

Pathogenesis

The development of a diseased or morbid condition.

Pathogens

An agent that causes disease, especially a living microorganism such as a bacterium, virus, or fungus.

Pathophysiology

The study of functional changes associated with or resulting from disease or injury.

PCR (Polymerase chain reaction)

A test used to detect extremely low quantities of pathogenic DNA or RNA, useful as a diagnosis and monitoring parameter of anti-pathogen treatment in LD. At present, the FDA has not yet endorsed it as a diagnostic method for LD.

Peripheral neuropathy

Disease or degenerative state of the peripheral nerves in which motor, sensory, or vasomotor nerve fibers may be affected and which is marked by muscle weakness and atrophy, pain, and numbness.

Peripheral neuritis

Inflammation of one or more peripheral nerves.

Phagocytosis

The engulfing and ingestion of bacteria or other foreign bodies by phagocytes, which are a kind of white blood cell.

Pharmacokinetics

The study of the process by which a drug is absorbed, distributed, metabolized, and eliminated by the body.

Phytochemical

Of or relating to phytochemistry, the study of the chemistry of plants.

Phytopharmacology

The study of the physiological actions of plant-based medicinal substances.

PMS (pre-menstrual syndrome)

A varied group of physical and psychological symptoms, including abdominal bloating, breast tenderness, headache, fatigue, irritability, anxiety, and depression, that occur from 2 to 7 days before the onset of menstruation and cease shortly after menses begins.

Positron emission computerized tomography (PET)

A computer-generated image of a biological activity within the body.

Prothrombin time

The time required for a particular specimen of prothrombin to induce blood-plasma clotting under standardized conditions in comparison with a time of between 11.5 and 12 seconds for normal human blood.

Protozoa

Any of a large group of single-celled, usually microscopic organisms, such as *amoebas, ciliates, flagellates,* and *sporozoans.*

Qi gong

An ancient Chinese system of postures, exercises, breathing techniques, and meditations to improve one's *qi* (*chi*), or energy field.

Raynaud's syndrome

A circulatory disorder that affects the hands and feet, caused by insufficient blood supply to these parts and resulting in cyanosis, numbness, pain, and, in extreme cases, gangrene.

Rat-bite fever

Either of two infectious diseases contractible from the bite of a rat, specifically, a disease caused by the *bacterium Streptobacillus moniliformis* and characterized by skin inflammation, back and joint pain, headache, and vomiting, or a disease caused by the *bacterium Spirillum* minus and characterized by ulceration at the site of the bite, a purplish rash, and recurrent fever.

Relapsing fever

Any of several infectious diseases characterized by chills and fever and caused by spirochetes transmitted by lice and ticks.

Rheumatoid arthritis

A chronic autoimmune disease marked by stiffness and inflammation of the joints, weakness, loss of mobility, and deformity.

Rocky Mountain fever

Also called Rocky Mountain spotted fever. A common co-infection of Lyme disease caused by infection of *Richettsia rickettsii*, transmitted by tick bite, and characterized by sudden onset of headache, chills, fever, and rashes.

Schistosomiasis

Various tropical diseases caused by infestation with *schistosomes*, widespread in rural areas of Africa, Asia, and Latin America through contact with contaminated water and characterized by gradual destruction of the kidneys, liver, and other organs. Also called bilharziasis or snail fever.

Sjogren syndrome

Chronic inflammatory autoimmune disease that particularly afflicts older women; is characterized by dryness of mucous membranes, especially of the eyes and mouth; and is often associated with rheumatoid arthritis.

SPECT scan

Single photon emission computerized tomography; a medical imaging technique that shows the functional activities of the brain.

Spheroplast

A bacterial cell whose cell wall is absent or deficient, causing it to have a spherical form.

Spirochete

Any of various slender, spiral, motile bacteria of the order *Spirochaetales*, many of which are pathogenic, causing syphilis, relapsing fever, yaws, and other diseases.

Syphilis

A chronic infectious disease caused by a spirochete (*Treponema pallidum*), either transmitted by direct contact, usually in sexual intercourse, or passed from mother to child in uterus.

Systematic lupus erythematosus (SLE)

A group of chronic autoimmune conditions characterized by skin lesions, congestion, edema, arthritis, and multiple organ damage.

Therapeutic index (Ld$_{50}$/ED$_{50}$)

The ratio between the toxic dose and the effective dose of a drug, used as a measure of its relative safety.

Tinnitus

A buzzing, ringing, or whistling in one or both ears that occurs without an external stimulus and is usually caused by an ear infection, the use of certain drugs, a blocked auditory tube or canal, or a head injury.

Toxoplasmosis

A disease caused by the sporozoan *Toxoplasma gondii* and characterized by lesions of the central nervous system that sometimes cause blindness and brain damage.

Trichomoniasis vaginitis

Acute or subacute vaginitis or urethritis caused by infection with the trichomonads *Trichomonas vaginalis*.

Tui-na

Chinese body work or massage.

Vasculitis

Inflammation of the blood vessels.

Vertigo

A sensation of irregular or whirling motion, either of oneself or of external objects.

Vasomotor mechanism

Relating to, causing, or regulating constriction or dilation of blood vessels.

Western blot

A laboratory test used for the detection of antibodies; a common diagnostic test for Lyme disease.

Yaws

An infectious disease caused by contact with the *bacterium Treponema pertenue* and with clinical manifestations that are similar to those for syphilis. Early treatment has high curative rate; late-stage patients may exhibit extensive deformities and dysfunctions.

Yin* and *yang

In Chinese philosophy, the two cosmic forces of creative energy, yin being feminine/negative and yang being masculine/positive, from which everything originates.

Zheng

TCM pattern of signs and symptoms of a disease or diseases.

Index

About the Author - Qingcai Zhang

Following graduation from Shanghai Second Medical University in 1962, Dr. Qingcai Zhang worked as a physician at the Medical University's Reijing Hospital, conducting clinical and laboratory research to integrate Chinese and Western medicine. He later became an associate professor of medicine at Shanghai Second Medical University.

In 1980, he was awarded a World Health Organization scholarship, which supported his two-year fellowship at Harvard Medical School and Massachusetts General Hospital. In 1984 he worked as a research fellow at the Wakai Clinic in Nagoya, Japan. A year later, he received a one-year appointment from the University of California at Davis as a visiting professor.

From 1986 to 1992, Dr. Zhang was the primary researcher at the Oriental Healing Arts Institute in Long Beach, California, where he conducted research on treating AIDS with Chinese medicine, designed herbal formulas for the treatment of AIDS, and published two books on AIDS and Chinese medicine.

He began his private practice in 1990, first in Cypress, California, and then in New York City. He is the founder of Zhang's Clinic in New York City and White Plains, New York. Since 1987, he has been focusing on treating chronic viral infections, such as viral hepatitis and AIDS; infectious diseases such as Lyme disease; and autoimmune diseases, such as inflammatory bowel disease, psoriasis, and rheumatoid arthritis.

Dr. Zhang is a member of the Hepatitis C Caring Ambassadors World Class Brainstorming Team, the Advisory Committee of the Science of Polaris Corporation, Dr. Weil's web site, and the Silvia Science Pharmaceutical Corporation. He has given lectures on modern Chinese medicine and AIDS, hepatitis, and Lyme disease nationwide.

Also by the author: AIDS and Chinese Medicine: Applications of the Oldest Medicine to the Newest Disease, Compound Q – Trichosanthin and its Clinical Applications, and Healing Hepatitis C with Modern Chinese Medicine. He is a contributing author of the following books: Hepatitis C Choices – Distinctive Viewpoints on Choices for Your Hepatitis C Journey, Alternative Medicine –The Definitive Guide, and Family Guide to Natural Medicine.

About the Co-Author - Yale Zhang

A graduate of the Wharton School of Finance, University of Pennsylvania, class of 2000, Yale Zhang received a bachelor's degree in economics and worked as a financial software developer for Argus Information and Advisory. He is the creator and moderator of Dr. Zhang's clinical websites, www.dr-zhang.com and www.sinomedresearch.org, and director of information technology at HepaPro Corporation. Currently, Yale is pursuing a post-graduate degree in Chinese medicine with the intention of continuing Dr. Zhang's research and clinical work.